Counseling in Speech-Language Pathology and Audiology

Reconstructing Personal Narratives

Counseling in Speech-Language Pathology and Audiology

Reconstructing Personal Narratives

Anthony DiLollo, PhD, CCC-SLP
Robert A. Neimeyer, PhD

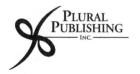

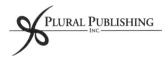
PLURAL PUBLISHING
INC.

5521 Ruffin Road
San Diego, CA 92123

e-mail: info@pluralpublishing.com
Web site: http://www.pluralpublishing.com

Copyright © by Plural Publishing, Inc. 2014

Typeset in 11/13 Garamond by Achorn International
Printed in the United States of America by McNaughton & Gunn, Inc.

FSC
www.fsc.org
MIX
Paper from
responsible sources
FSC® C011935

Cover image: *Untitled,* watercolor and pen and ink by David Acevedo. Copyright ©2003 Robert Neimeyer.

Library of Congress Cataloging-in-Publication Data

DiLollo, Anthony, author.
    Counseling in speech-language pathology and audiology : reconstructing personal narratives / Anthony DiLollo, Robert A. Neimeyer.
        p. ; cm.
    Includes bibliographical references and index.
    ISBN 978-1-59756-484-7 (alk. paper)
    ISBN 1-59756-484-2 (alk. paper)
    I. Neimeyer, Robert A., 1954– author.   II. Title.
    [DNLM: 1. Communication Disorders—therapy. 2. Counseling—methods.
    3. Narrative Therapy. 4. Personal Construct Theory. WM 475]
    RC428.8
    616.85'506—dc23
                                                                    2014005090

CONTENTS

FOREWORD

It is a pleasure to be asked to prepare a foreword for any good book. But it is a special pleasure to do so when you are familiar with the authors' work and look forward to reading chapters that you know will be thoughtfully and skillfully prepared. Students and professional clinicians in the professions of speech-language pathology and audiology will find this book an essential tool in their therapeutic practice. As I read through the concise and engaging chapters, I often found myself thinking of the many clinicians who—as the research indicates—are hesitant about counseling their clients. Although all readers and their clients will benefit from this book, it is the hesitant clinicians who will find this book especially useful. DiLollo and Neimeyer provide the clinician with a clear theoretical rationale and intuitively appealing processes for connecting with and assisting clients with communication problems. Readers will be moved by the case illustrations that document the heroic journeys that are possible as a result of effective counseling for communication problems.

The authors explain in the preface that their goal in writing this book is "to provide an empirically informed and practically oriented manual for counseling clients with a broad range of communication disorders" (p. X). Their many years of counseling experience are necessary for achieving this goal. But it's their thoughtful sequencing of the 26 chapters and their clear and engaging writing style that make it happen.

The early chapters provide a model that includes counseling as a natural and essential feature of the therapeutic experience for those with communication problems. The authors also document that counseling is clearly within the scope of practice for professionals in our discipline and that effective therapy and counseling are inseparable. They make the essential point that, in the vast majority of cases, we are assisting essentially healthy people who must cope with specific communication problems rather than people who need help with more basic personality issues. Of the four levels of progressively more concentrated counseling outlined in Chapter 2, the first two levels of counseling, focusing on a greater understanding of the client's situation and the client's ability to experiment and adapt to more effective coping, are all that is necessary for most individuals.

In Chapter 3, the authors describe the unique stance of the clinician as one of "adaptive leadership" rather than providing a service intended to "fix" the client. Rather than considering the person through the lens of the medical model where a breakdown in the system needs to be repaired, a more holistic approach is offered that considers the person as a complex adaptive system where changes to one part of the system results in changes to other parts. The primary goal of the clinician is to mobilize the client to do the work that is necessary for change to occur. Adaptive leadership by the clinician leads to adaptive change by the clients, with clients experimenting, not only with new ways of behaving, but also with new ways of conceptualizing themselves and their situations. In this chapter and throughout the book, the authors provide vivid examples of clinical experiences that illustrate the concepts and techniques that are necessary for change.

Part II (Chapters 4–8) provides clear descriptions of the theoretical foundations of counseling (humanistic therapy, behavior therapy, and cognitive therapy) and introduces the reader to the primary focus of the book, the constructivist-narrative approach. Part III (Chapters 9–13) describes the processes that are part of the constructivist-narrative approach, with each process accompanied by a case description that is both vivid and moving.

The reader begins to appreciate that at the core of the constructivist-narrative approach is a focus on the "client as the expert" and each client's personal narrative. Rather than being in the role of the expert or the "fixer," the clinician has the opportunity to share an adventure with clients as they alter their relationship with their problems. The clinician's stance is that of a curious observer and listener of the client's current narrative. As the client's dominant narrative is deconstructed and externalized via activities that are a natural part of the therapeutic conversation, the conceptualization of the situation moves from "the person as the problem" to "the problem as the problem." The therapeutic experience becomes more about the development of a dynamic therapeutic alliance and the meaning of the activities as much or more than it is about the behavioral techniques that are a necessary but not a sufficient aspect of successful therapeutic change. The goal is to help clients to experiment with their relationship with the problem and to develop an agentic life style. Along with providing supporting empirical evidence for the effectiveness of the constructivist-narrative approach, the case illustrations in Chapters 11 and 12 bring home informative and touching examples of the power of adaptive counseling centered on the client and client's resources and values.

Part IV (Chapters 14–25) describes the rationale and procedures associated with a variety of "tools" for working with clients from the constructivist-narrative perspective. These 12 chapters in Part IV are intended to be stand-alone chapters that can be read by the clinician as the need arises. The final section (Part V, Chapter 26) is a thoughtful addition intended to help instructors teach the constructivist counseling framework to students.

As a clinician and a person with a history of stuttering, I have often witnessed two essential changes that occur during a successful therapy experience—clients' abilities to reconstruct their cognitive view of themselves and to successfully manage their communication problem. This book provides a concise, engaging, and effective way for the client and the clinician to facilitate those changes and create an agentic and autonomous lifestyle. I recommend it to both students in the discipline and seasoned professionals who are looking for a theoretically elegant, empirically informed, and immensely practical way of helping clients revise constraining stories of their relationship to their communication problems in the course of responsive counseling.

—Walter H. Manning, PhD
Professor, School of Communication Sciences and Disorders
The University of Memphis
Author of: *Clinical Decision Making in Fluency Disorders*
Clifton Park, NY: Delmar | Cengage Learning
March 2014

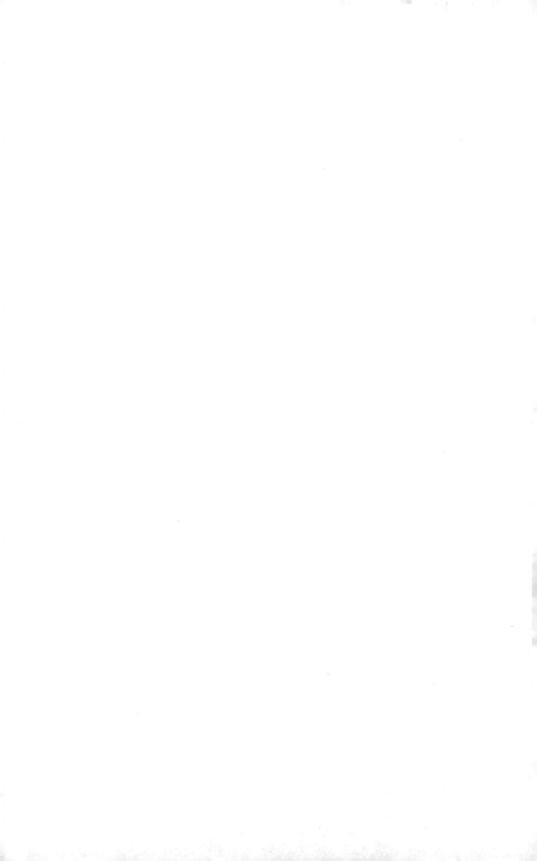

PREFACE

This book arises from the convergence of life experiences within us as professionals in different disciplines, and between us in dialogue across 15 years of collaboration. Before delving into the principles and practices that inform the approach to counseling in the fields of speech-language pathology (SLP) and audiology represented in these pages, we thought it would be useful to give readers a sense of where we are "coming from," so that they can better anticipate what they are "headed toward" in the chapters to come. What follows, then, is basically an abridged story of how this unusual book came to be. For clarity, and to anticipate the focus on dialogue that informs our approach to counseling, we will tell the story as a conversation or interview between the first author, Tony DiLollo, and second author, Bob Neimeyer.

Bob: Why don't you get it started, Tony. How did you come to hatch the idea of a novel book on counseling in your field in the first place?

Tony: Well, Bob, my interest in counseling in speech-language pathology really started with my connection with my first real mentor, Dr. Thomas A. Crowe, at the University of Mississippi. Tom was an accomplished practitioner and researcher in the area of fluency disorders, but also a psychologist by training and counselor by nature. Noting my psychology and counseling background—as I had worked for some years as a school counselor in Fremantle, the port town of Perth, Western Australia—he took me under his wing and started me on my way as a speech-language pathologist who regarded counseling as a central tenet of our profession. In 1996, as Dr. Crowe's Graduate Assistant, I spent many enjoyable hours assisting him in putting together his textbook on counseling,

Applications of Counseling in Speech-Language Pathology and Audiology, learning not just about counseling, but also about the creative process and the time, commitment, and desire that go into tackling such a project. In the process of writing, now, our own book on counseling in speech-language pathology and audiology, I have often reflected on those experiences many years ago in Oxford.

Bob: Yes, I recall meeting you not long after you ventured north to Memphis after your time in Oxford, as you completed your program there and entered doctoral training here. Looking back at that shift, how did your early interest in counseling in SLP that germinated at Ole Miss begin to grow into the concept of a book project during your Memphis years?

Tony: Good question. I'd say there were three driving forces behind the writing of this book, the first being my belief that counseling should be an underlying tenet of the practice of speech-language pathology and audiology. This belief, of course, has been echoed by many over the years but was personalized for me through my clinical experiences and the mentorship, first of Tom Crowe, and then, as I began my doctoral studies at the University of Memphis, of Dr. Walt Manning in the speech-language pathology field and Dr. David Wark in audiology. As I continued working and studying, I recognized a growing sense that, as a speech-language pathologist, treating merely the problem, rather than the person, represented a fundamental flaw in our approach to clinical practice and left many clients experiencing little to no improvement in quality of life, despite technical improvement in their speech or language problem.

The second driving force behind the writing of this book has been my belief that a constructivist approach to counseling is particularly well suited to the work we do as speech-language pathologists and audiologists. Early in my doctoral program, I was fortunate enough to encounter *constructivism* as reflected in some preliminary work that David Wark had done with you in the Psychology Department at the University of Memphis. At his urging, I enthusiastically enrolled in several of your courses, marinating myself deeply in the person-centered, meaning-based approach to therapy that you taught. As I learned about constructivism and began investigating its applications to various personal and behavioral problems, I began to recognize how applicable the approach might be in helping people with communication disorders.

Bob: I have to say that I remember your engagement in those classes fondly, even after 15 years! Not only could I count on you to keep the psychology doctoral students on their toes in class discussion, but you also opened the door to a long series of audiology and SLP students in those same courses: Rebecca Kelly, Kyunjae Lee, Katie Shaughnessy, Laura Plexico, Janice Tanedo, and others. Like you, and like Walt and Dave, they seemed to get bitten by the constructivist bug and naturally began incorporating narrative and meaning-oriented practices into their counseling with SLP and audiology clients. Some even went on to do significant research in the area, as we discuss in later chapters. But you seemed to take it a step further, and launched a whole series of studies bringing constructivist methods and insights to bear on questions in your field. How did that happen?

Tony: Well, we all have to complete a dissertation! But in all seriousness, it seemed natural to me to propose and test some of the implications of this type of counseling with persons with communication disorders. I remember that the work of Fay Fransella from back in the 1970's with persons who stutter really got me excited, as she put into practice many of the thoughts that I had been having in your classes! Then I came across the narrative therapy work of Michael White (an Aussie, by the way!) and the concept of counseling through conversations rather than "techniques" just seemed like such a natural fit for what we do in communication disorders. As a result, during my doctoral studies, you probably remember that I developed a "workbook" to be used with persons who stutter. It was designed to facilitate constructivist counseling-type conversations to help clinicians engage clients in counseling. In many ways, that workbook was the precursor to a series of peer-reviewed journal articles as well as to the book that we are now introducing.

The third driving force behind the writing of this book actually began percolating many years ago when I was working as a school counselor in a small, private middle and high school in that port town back in Australia. Despite gaining a Psychology degree from the University of Western Australia that included numerous hours of coursework becoming familiar with a myriad of different approaches to psychotherapy, in practice I felt like I was working in the dark. It wasn't until some years later—I was by then practicing as a speech-language pathologist in the United States—that I realized that what I was missing was an organizing framework on which to base my counseling efforts. What I needed was a way to consistently conceptualize the people and problems that I was being asked to help with. When I started teaching counseling to speech-language pathology and audiology students, I realized that if I simply provided them with the standard overview of approaches to counseling that typically form the core of counseling courses in our field, they were going to have no more clarity about the process of engaging clients than I had as a school counselor. Consequently, I began to focus on helping students build a constructivist counseling framework that would aid them in understanding clients and their problems. I have spent more than 10 years teaching this framework to speech-language pathology and audiology students, first at Ole Miss, and now at Wichita State University in Kansas, and ultimately this is what gave rise to the idea of writing a theoretically enlightened, empirically informed, and practically oriented manual for counseling clients with a broad range of communication disorders. The goal of this book, therefore, was not to provide techniques for counseling, nor was it to set out a prescriptive method of "doing" counseling. Instead, the goal of this book is to help students and clinicians develop *a way of thinking* that guides them in interpreting clients' behaviors and understanding clients' problems from the perspective of the clients themselves. By thinking in terms of clients' personal stories and the impact that those stories have on their communication difficulties, I've found that students and supervisees are able to implement the treatments that we provide as communication specialists much more effectively. By doing so, clinicians can empower clients to find the personal resources and strengths to generate solutions to their own problems and reconstruct preferred identities out of stories of disability.

Bob: That makes a native kind of sense to me, of course. As a constructivist psychologist who has engaged in both research and practice on a weekly basis for 30 years—including working with people who present with problems of speech and hearing alongside other life challenges—I obviously join you in believing in counseling as an empowering practice. That is what has made the project of this book surprisingly easy, moving from our collaborative research to the conceptualization of constructivist counseling as a form of *leadership*, and from setting out a "toolkit" of creative practices to illustrating them in specific case studies. I also fully join you in hoping that the ideas outlined in these pages will help clients in your field find their own voice in the midst of the often silencing and isolating presence of their problems.

Tony: Well said. We both hope that the chapters that follow will inspire readers to experiment with novel procedures, and in a sense to read between the lines of the client's story of brokenness and deficiency to see the seeds of resilience that can be nurtured by counseling. To sum it up, I believe that infusing counseling for speech-language pathology and audiology with constructivist and narrative practices can enhance the benefits and "staying power" of the more technical interventions also utilized in therapy.

Bob: Spoken like a true constructivist! Let the story begin!

—Anthony DiLollo, PhD, Wichita State University and
Robert A. Neimeyer, PhD, University of Memphis
January 2014

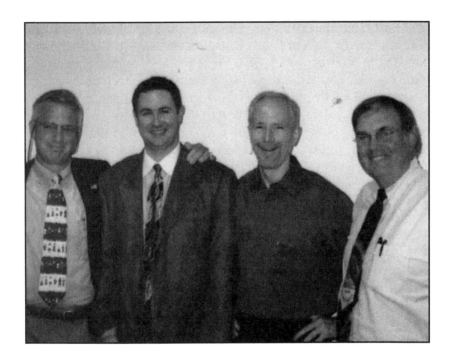

ACKNOWLEDGMENTS

Every writer of every book accumulates a substantial debt, both intellectual and personal. In our case, we are indebted to the intellectual mentors we came to know through their printed word— George Kelly, the author of personal construct theory; Carl Rogers, originator of person-centered therapy; and a pantheon of other authors whose writing inspires our own. Equally, we owe more than we can acknowledge to those mentors and colleagues we have known in the flesh—Michael White and David Epston, founders of the narrative therapy model much in evidence in these pages; Fay Fransella, who first bridged the gulf separating the field of communication disorders from that of clinical psychology; and others named and unnamed in the chapters that follow. Most specifically, we want to salute those teachers, colleagues, and friends who helped us appreciate the central role of constructive counseling in the fields of speech-language pathology and audiology—Tom Crowe, Walt Manning, Chris Constantino, and David and Marilyn Wark. Without their encouragement and often co-authorship, the present project would not have found the fertile conceptual soil needed to put down roots, grow, and ultimately bear fruit. To all of these colleagues, living and dead, we tip our *akubra* hats in a grateful salute.

Likewise, and still more personally, we appreciate the unflagging support of our families, and most especially our wives, Lara and Kathy, for tolerating the multiple "working vacations" in which one of us stayed in the "Garage Mahal" guest quarters behind the other's home, as we labored like 21st century monastic scribes on our Apple computers to produce and revise many of the chapters that constitute the present volume. For their patience and willingness to pick up the slack during the innumerable additional hours we spent in solitary writing and e-mail correspondence, we owe them more than the obligatory celebratory dinner when the book hits print.

We also owe a debt of thanks to Milgem Rabanera—or Gem, as we have come to know her—and her colleagues at Plural Publishing for their support throughout this process. In our endeavor to create a book that not only informed but also reflected constructivist and narrative practices, we often seemed to be stepping outside the "norms" for textbooks in communication disorders. Gem's patience and guidance were invaluable in helping us reach our destination.

Also, to Imran Musaji, who read versions of many chapters and worked diligently on the arduous tasks of proofing and indexing, we thank you—we could not have asked for a better graduate assistant to help with this project.

And finally, we want to thank the many clients whose stories are told or implied in the succeeding chapters, and the many students who have shared them in classrooms and supervision, while adding clinical accounts of their own. With both the protagonists of these stories of counseling and with their audience, we have discovered and rediscovered the power of narrative to inspire clinical creativity and transform lives. We hope that in its own way the current book contributes to this process for readers and the clients alongside of whom they work.

—Tony DiLollo and Bob Neimeyer

CONTRIBUTOR

Christopher D. Constantino, MS
School of Communication Sciences and Disorders
University of Memphis
Memphis, Tennessee
Chapters 20, 21, 22, and 25

To Lara
You are my Muse
AD

To clinical pioneers in all fields
For crossing the frontiers that separate us
RAN

Part I

GETTING ORIENTED

The three chapters in Part I are designed to help readers get oriented to the concept of counseling in speech-language pathology and audiology and to help them differentiate between technical and adaptive aspects of clients' problems.

1

COUNSELING IN COMMUNICATION DISORDERS

What is the role of counseling when working with people who have communication disorders? The answer, it seems, depends on who you ask! On the one hand, the official position of the American Speech-Language-Hearing Association (ASHA) and the American Academy of Audiology (AAA) is to regard it as a mandatory dimension of clinical practice, as we will see below. On the other hand, more than a few students and practitioners are leery of stepping into a territory they associate more with psychology or psychiatry than with speech-language pathology or audiology. Our goal in this brief chapter is to provide a general introduction to the concept of counseling in our fields by exploring the "disconnect" between policy and practice, and to consider prevalent myths about clinical practice that act as barriers to counseling.

> *A number of years ago, I was teaching a course on counseling to speech-language pathology and audiology graduate students. We had just finished a discussion of the importance of counseling and the need to get to know your client's story when, during a break, one of the students came up to talk with me. "I have an aphasia client," she said, "and, based on*

what we have been learning in this class, I wanted to spend our first session together getting to know her and how she feels about her life now." "That sounds like a great idea," I said, feeling rather pleased with myself for making an impact—until she finished her story: "But my supervisor told me that I had to follow my lesson plan because the client came here for therapy, not counseling."

A Mandate for Counseling

As speech-language pathologists and audiologists, what we do is at least in part directed by a series of documents that have been carefully drafted by committees of our peers through our national accrediting agencies, ASHA and AAA. These documents provide detailed descriptions of the role of speech-language pathologists and audiologists, including the skills and practice patterns that are deemed appropriate given the goals of the professions.

Scope of Practice and Preferred Practice Patterns

The term "counseling" is specifically and extensively referenced in key documents officially regulating practice for both speech-language pathology and audiology. For example, in the *ASHA Scope of Practice for Speech-Language Pathology* (ASHA, 2007), the wording related to counseling clearly states that clinicians should engage in "counseling individuals, families, coworkers, educators, and other persons in the community regarding acceptance, adaptation, and decision making about communication and swallowing." Furthermore, ASHA's document titled *Preferred Practice Patterns for the Profession of Speech-Language Pathology* (ASHA, 2004) notes that counseling should be "conducted by appropriately credentialed and trained speech-language pathologists" and that it should involve "providing timely information and guidance to patients/clients, families/caregivers, and other relevant persons about the nature of communication or swallowing disorders, the course of intervention, ways to enhance outcomes, coping with disorders, and prognosis."

Similarly, ASHA's *Scope of Practice for Audiology* (ASHA, 2003) specifically mentions counseling in its description of "what audiologists do," and *The Preferred Practice Patterns for the Profession of Audiology* (ASHA, 2006) lists counseling in Section IV, Item 23, and provides a detailed description of the process of counseling as "interactive and facilitative, wherein the communicative, psychosocial, and behavioral adjustment problems associated with auditory, vestibular, or other related disorders can be ameliorated." Furthermore, AAA's *Scope of Practice* (AAA, 2004) document describes the role of the audiologist as providing "counseling regarding the effects of hearing loss on communication and psychosocial status in personal, social, and vocational arenas." Likewise, AAA's *Standards of Practice for Audiology* (AAA, 2012) indicates that audiologists must provide counseling to "improve a person's use of residual auditory and/or vestibular function or cope with the consequences of a loss of function" and to "provide support to patients and their caregivers to address the potential psychosocial impact of auditory and vestibular deficits."

In addition to scope of practice and preferred practice patterns, both AAA and ASHA provide a code of ethics that also guide clinicians in what they do. Both of these Code of Ethics documents (AAA, 2011; ASHA, 2010) mandate that clinicians should engage in all aspects of the professions within the scope of practice and provide all services competently, using all available resources to provide high-quality service.

What emerges from study of these guiding documents is that we as clinicians have a mandate to provide clinical services beyond the simple teaching of behavioral techniques or use of technology. Moreover, it is our ethical responsibility to seek further education to ensure that we are providing services commensurate with our scope of practice and preferred practice patterns.

A Disconnect Between Principles and Clinical Practice

As might be gleaned from the vignette at the start of this chapter, despite the clear mandate to engage in counseling embodied in the scope of practice and preferred practice patterns for both audiology and speech-language pathology, many clinicians historically have been reluctant to provide such services (Citron, 2000; Clark, 1994; Crowe, 1997; Erdman, 2000; Garstecki & Erler, 1997; Kendall, 2000; Luterman, 2001; Rollin, 2000; Stone & Olswang, 1989; Sweetow, 1999). More recently, Holland (2007) and Simmons-Mackie and Damico (2011) reaffirm this reluctance, reporting that speech-language pathologists continue to resist engaging clients in a counseling relationship. Silverman (2011) further suggests that many speech-language pathologists in the United States believe that counseling is simply not a part their job description. With a certain degree of cynicism, Silverman states that these clinicians prefer to think of themselves more akin to physicians, even adopting the medical title of "pathologist." She warns, however, that, "it is well to remember that physicians who practice pathology study the causes, nature, and effects of diseases by examining organs, tissues, fluids, and dead bodies. They do not relate to living patients. Assuming the mantle of speech-language pathologist has led many of us to practice similarly" (p. 190). Why, then, does this disconnect between our guiding principles and clinical practice exist? To consider this question, in the next section we will address some of the myths about clinical practice that seem to act as barriers to clinicians engaging in counseling.

Myths About Clinical Practice

Through both anecdotal evidence from clinicians and a more formal review of the literature, several possible explanations emerge for why clinicians in our field fail to engage in counseling in their clinical practice. In this section, we look at a few of the common "myths" that militate against audiologists and speech-language pathologists engaging in counseling, and how the current text might provide clinicians with the necessary tools to overcome these barriers.

   Myth #1: Behavioral principles are sufficient. Behavioral treatment methods are typically very good at addressing surface behaviors and symptoms but are less well suited to addressing deeper issues that relate to the emotional and psychosocial consequences of communication disorders. Of particular difficulty for behavioral methods is promoting long-term, meaningful change, as is evident from the high rates of relapse for strictly behavioral treatments of addictive disorders (Craig, 1998) and stuttering (Craig & Hancock, 1995).

The framework for counseling described in this book is designed to complement rather than replace traditional behavioral approaches to treatment in speech-language pathology to allow clinicians to impact both psychosocial/emotional and behavioral aspects of communication disorders.

Myth #2: Counseling is the province of psychologists and counselors, not speech-language pathologists or audiologists. The World Health Organization's (WHO) health classification system, known as the International Classification of Functioning, Disability, and Health (ICF; WHO, 2001), forms the framework for ASHA's preferred practice patterns and scope of practice for both audiology and speech-language pathology. This classification system proposes that disorders—including speech, language, swallowing, and hearing disorders—consist of more than the simple observable behavioral and structural disruptions, giving equal status to more intrinsic aspects related to attitudes, psychosocial, and emotional factors. Given this approach to classifying disorders, speech-language pathologists and audiologists are reminded that their treatment of speech, language, swallowing, or hearing disorders must address these less concrete factors; and the only effective method for doing so is through engaging clients in counseling.

The framework for counseling described in this book has been designed specifically with audiologists and speech-language pathologists in mind. It is based in established psychotherapeutic theory and practice but tailored to fit the unique demands that speech-language pathologists and audiologists face in their clinical practices and to seamlessly merge with many of the behavioral activities that clinicians are already using.

Myth #3: Contemporary clinical practice has advanced to the point where addressing the human side of the problem is no longer necessary. Just as with other areas of knowledge, clinical practice in our field has improved over the past

50 years. Advances in pharmaceutical, genetic, prosthetic, and technological treatments for disorders continue to rapidly alter the landscape of clinical practice in many fields. Although this may be true for some areas of audiology and speech-language pathology such as hearing-aid technology, cochlear implants, augmentative and alternative communication devices, and tracheoesophageal puncture surgery, to name a few, there remains a "human" element to any aspect of treatment for communication disorders. The fundamental goal of clinical practice in our fields remains "improved quality of life" for our clients (ASHA, 2004, 2006), and, to that end, clients need support and guidance in order to adapt to the advanced treatment methods or technology provided to them by clinicians.

The goal of the framework for counseling described in this book is to provide a way for clinicians to conceptualize clients and their problems at a meaningful level in order to facilitate improvements in their quality of life.

Myth #4: In the current managed care environment, clinicians do not have time for counseling. This is not so much a myth as it is a misunderstanding of what it takes to engage clients in counseling. Certainly, in today's managed care environment, and even in other environments such as schools, speech-language pathologists and audiologists are expected to deal with high caseloads and rapid turnaround times between appointments. Clinicians therefore can conclude that they simply don't have time to add counseling to what they already do. Fortunately, effective counseling can take place through simply recognizing a client's anxiety, acknowledging a client's choices, and engaging clients' in even very brief conversations that tell their story. Sometimes clients may be engaged in counseling simply by adjusting the way an existing activity has always been done. At other times, inviting clients to reflect on their experience with treatment between appointments can improve the outcome of therapy, while requiring very little additional time on the part of the clinician. Furthermore, investing some time at the front end of assessment or treatment can pay off later through greater "compliance" and satisfaction on the part of the client.

The purpose of this book is to provide clinicians with a framework for engaging clients in counseling that will not necessarily add significantly to the time spent with each client and will help clinicians recognize opportunities to counsel simply by being genuine, interested, conversational partners.

Myth #5: Only objective, measurable procedures with established empirical evidence should be used in clinical practice; other procedures are unscientific and invalid. This myth stems from a misunderstanding of evidence-based practice (EBP) and what it has to say about appropriate evidence for different types of treatment. To begin with, numerous authors (e.g., Botterill, 2011; Horvath, 2001; Luterman, 2001; Manning, 2010; Wampold, 2001) have documented the importance of the therapeutic alliance across a great range of counseling approaches. In fact, Wampold reports that the quality of the relationship between counselor and client accounts for a significantly greater proportion of therapeutic change than do the specific types of treatment. These findings provide evidence for engaging in counseling with clients and suggest that, regardless of the specific "technical" approach that clinicians implement, taking the time to engage the client in a counseling relationship is likely to produce the most effective treatment.

Second, according to ASHA (2005), EBP is "an approach in which current, high-quality research evidence is integrated with practitioner expertise and the individual's preferences and values into the process of clinical decision making" (p. 1). Dollaghan (2004), however, points out that some parts of this definition (i.e., the "current, high-quality research evidence") tend to receive more attention than others and that "practitioner expertise" and "individual's preferences and values" should be considered equally when making clinical decisions. Similarly, Ratner (2006) suggests that, when applying EBP to speech-language pathology, questions must be raised regarding linking outcomes to treatments. For example, if treatment outcomes are favorable, was it the therapy or the therapist that accounted for the effect? Manning (2010) also points out that, when the implications of EBP for clinical decision-making are being considered, care should be taken to distinguish between an approach that is empirically unvalidated (i.e., not enough data to make a decision) and one that is empirically invalidated (i.e., data indicate that the treatment is not efficacious). Although the latter should be ruled out as a treatment option, the former might well be included, especially if, in the judgment of the clinician, it could enhance or reinforce the value of an evidence-based procedure.

In short, the counseling framework described in this book: (a) is compatible with basic constructivist research in communication disorders, reviewed in Chapter 7, (b) is based on widely researched and applied psychotherapeutic approaches, and (c) is focused on building the therapeutic alliance through attention to the client's personal story. By clearly conveying specific methods and techniques in Part IV of this book, we also invite researchers to further evaluate their impact in improving clinical outcomes in our field.

Myth #6: Training in the communication disorders disciplines is insufficient to permit competent practice in counseling. Unfortunately, authors from both speech-language pathology and audiology (e.g., Crandell, 1997; Culpepper, Mendel, & McCarthy, 1994; Flasher & Fogle, 2004; Kaderavek, Laux, & Mills 2004; Kendall, 2000; Luterman, 2001; McCarthy, Culpepper, & Lucks, 1986) have pointed out that inadequate training and preparation of clinicians in the area of counseling remains a primary barrier to more widespread use of counseling in communication disorders. For example, McCarthy, et al. found that coursework in counseling was required in only 33% of programs accredited by ASHA at that time and only 12% of students believed that they had been adequately prepared to engage clients in counseling. More recently, Luterman (2008) and Phillips and Mendel (2008) arrived at similar conclusions, indicating that little had changed in the 20 years since McCarthy, et al.'s study.

The purpose of this book is to provide both students and professional clinicians with a contemporary framework for counseling that is effective but relatively easy to start using. As clinicians begin to apply the framework to their own everyday experiences as well as to their clinical experiences (remember, life experience prepares you for counseling!) they should find it easier and more intuitive, as it becomes a trustworthy way of thinking rather than a set of rules or procedures to follow.

Myth #7: I don't know when to do counseling and when to do traditional therapy. Thinking of counseling in this way is like suggesting that you need to set aside a specific time to 'show affection' to your partner. In most cases, counseling with speech-language pathology or audiology clients is not something that is put on the lesson plan! With a few exceptions, there is no need to schedule a specific time for counseling. Rather, it is something that happens as clinicians react to the client as a person (rather than as a speech, language, swallowing, or hearing problem), and is integrally woven into the traditional therapy or assessment activities that clinicians already perform.

The framework for counseling presented in this book was designed to be integrated into the existing clinical practices of audiologists and speech-language pathologists. Chapter 3 in this text is also designed to help clinicians identify the technical aspects of a client's problem (those aspects that require technical expertise such as certain treatment or technological approaches) and the adaptive aspects (those that suggest more of a counseling approach). Seen in this light, technique and counseling are not so much competitive as complementary.

Conclusion

Counseling is an integral component of any treatment and something that all speech-language pathologists and audiologists should be engaged in—at some level—with all of their clients. It is within the scope of practice for both disciplines, as well as part of the preferred practice patterns and ethical obligations for clinicians as determined by AAA and ASHA. Despite this, there is often reluctance on the part of some clinicians to engage in this practice, often due to myths and misperceptions about counseling itself and clinical practice in general.

Our goal in this book is to help close the gap between principles and practice by building a bridge between clinicians' intent and capacity. In the next chapter we discuss how this book can be used to support both novice and experienced clinicians who are striving to augment their effectiveness within the scope of practice of their profession. Let's get started!

References

American Academy of Audiology. (2004). *Scope of practice.* Retrieved September 29, 2013, from http://www.audiology.org/resources/document library/Pages/ScopeofPractice.aspx

American Academy of Audiology. (2011). *Code of ethics*. Retrieved September 29, 2013, from http://www.audiology.org/resources/document library/Pages/codeofethics.aspx

American Academy of Audiology. (2012). *Standards of practice for audiology*. Retrieved September 29, 2013, from http://www.audiology.org /resources/documentlibrary/Pages/StandardsofPractice.aspx

American Speech-Language-Hearing Association. (2003). *Scope of practice audiology*. Rockville, MD: Author.

American Speech-Language-Hearing Association. (2004). *Preferred practice patterns for the profession of speech-language pathology*. Rockville, MD: Author.

American Speech-Language-Hearing Association. (2005). *Evidence-based practice in communication disorders* [Position statement]. Retrieved from http://www.asha.org/policy.

American Speech-Language-Hearing Association. (2006). *Preferred practice patterns for the profession of audiology*. Rockville, MD: Author.

American Speech-Language-Hearing Association. (2007). *Scope of practice in speech-language pathology*. Rockville, MD: Author.

American Speech-Language-Hearing Association. (2010). *Code of ethics* [Ethics]. Retrieved from http://www.asha.org/policy.

Botterill, W. (2011). Developing the therapeutic relationship: From "expert" professional to "expert" person who stutters. *Journal of Fluency Disorders, 36*, 158–173.

Citron III, D. (2000). Counseling and orientation toward amplification. In M. Valente, H. Hosford-Dunn, & R. J. Roeser (Eds.), *Audiology treatment*. New York, NY: Thieme Medical Publishers, Inc.

Clark, J. G. (1994). Understanding, building and maintaining relationships with patients. In J. G. Clark & F. N. Martin (Eds.), *Effective counseling in audiology*. Englewood Cliffs, NJ: Prentice Hall.

Craig, A. (1998). Relapse following treatment for stuttering: A critical review and correlative data. *Journal of Fluency Disorders, 23*, 1–30.

Craig, A. R., & Hancock, K. (1995). Self-reported factors related to relapse following treatment for stuttering. *Australian Journal of Human Communication Disorders, 23*, 48–60.

Crandell, C. C. (1997). An update on counseling instruction within audiology programs. *Journal of Audiological Rehabilitation Association, 30*, 77–86.

Crowe, T. A. (Ed.) (1997). *Applications of counseling in speech-language pathology and audiology*. Philadelphia, PA: Williams & Wilkins.

Culpepper, B., Lucks Mendel, L., & McCarthy, P. A. (1994). Counseling experience and training offered by ESB-accredited programs. *ASHA, 36*, 55–58.

Dollaghan, C. (2004, April 13). Evidence-based practice: Myths and realities. *The ASHA Leader*, pp. 4-5, 12.

Erdman, S. A. (2000). Counseling adults with hearing impairment. In J. G. Alpiner & P. A. McCarthy (Eds.), *Rehabilitative audiology children and adults* (3rd ed.). Baltimore, MD: Lippincott Williams & Wilkins.

Flasher, L., & Fogle, P. (2004). *Counseling skills for the speech-language pathologist and audiologist.* Clifton Park, NY: Thomson-Delmar Learning.

Garstecki, D. C., & Erler, S. F. (1997). Counseling older adult hearing instrument candidates. *Hearing Review Supplement, 1,* 14-18.

Holland, A. (2007). *Counseling in communication disorders: A wellness perspective.* San Diego, CA: Plural.

Horvath, A. O. (2001). The therapeutic alliance: Concepts, research, and training. *Australian Psychologist, 36,* 170-176.

Kaderavek, J. N., Laux, J. M., & Mills, N. H. (2004). A counseling training module for students in speech-language pathology training programs. *Contemporary Issues in Communication Science and Disorders, 31,* 153-161.

Kendall, D. L. (2000). Counseling in communication disorders. *Contemporary Issues in Communication Science and Disorders, 27,* 96-103.

Luterman, D. M. (2001). *Counseling persons with communication disorders and their families.* (4th Ed.), Austin, TX: Pro-Ed, Inc.

Luterman, D. M. (2008). *Counseling persons with communication disorders and their families.* (5th Ed.), Austin, TX: Pro-Ed, Inc.

Manning, W. H. (2010). *Clinical decision making in fluency disorders* (3rd ed.). Clifton Park, NY: Delmar, Cengage Learning.

McCarthy, P. A., Culpepper, B., & Lucks, L. (1986). Variability in counseling experiences and training among ESB accredited programs. *ASHA, 28,* 49-52.

Phillips, D., & Mendel, L. (2008). Counseling training in communication disorders: A survey of clinical fellows. *Contemporary Issues in Communication Science and Disorders, 35,* 44-53.

Ratner, N. B. (2006). Evidence-based practice: An examination of its ramifications for the practice of speech-language pathology. *Language, Speech, & Hearing Services in Schools, 37,* 257-267.

Rollin, W. J. (2000). *Counseling individuals with communication disorders: Psychodynamic and family aspects* (2nd ed.). Boston, MA: Butterworth-Heinemann.

Silverman, E. M. (2011). Self-reflection in clinical practice (pp. 183-193). In R. J. Fourie (Ed.), *Therapeutic processes for communication disorders: A guide for clinicians and students.* New York, NY: Psychology Press.

Simmons-Mackie, N., & Damico, J. S. (2011). Counseling and aphasia treatment: Missed opportunities. *Topics in Language Disorders, 31,* 336–351.

Stone, J. R., & Olswang, L. B. (1989). The hidden challenge in counseling. *ASHA, 31,* 27–31.

Sweetow, R. W. (1999). Counseling: The secret to successful hearing aid fittings. In R. W. Sweetow (Ed.), *Counseling for hearing aid fittings.* San Diego, CA: Singular Publishing Group.

Wampold, B. E. (2001). *The great psychotherapy debate: Models, methods, and findings.* Mahwah, NJ: Lawrence Erlbaum Associates.

World Health Organization. (2002). *International Classification of Functioning, Disability and Health.* Geneva, Switzerland: Author.

2

WHAT DOES COUNSELING REALLY MEAN FOR SPEECH-LANGUAGE PATHOLOGISTS AND AUDIOLOGISTS?

It seemed like a relatively straightforward exercise. "Write about an experience of loss" were the basic instructions from my professor, Dr. Neimeyer. I was just starting out in a doctoral program in Audiology and Speech-Language Pathology (AUSP) at the University of Memphis and was enrolled in a "constructivist psychotherapy" course that had been recommended by an AUSP faculty member. I chose to write about the loss of my grandfather some 20 years earlier. I took the assignment seriously and wrote at length about my feelings of loss at the time and how they continued into the present, with real regret that my grandfather never got to know me as an adult. I submitted the assignment and received a pleasing grade with positive comments from

15

Dr. Neimeyer. A few weeks later, my wife and I were to leave town, leaving our two young boys at home with my in-laws, to fly to San Francisco for a professional conference. As the time approached, I began to feel a rising apprehension that quickly turned into outright fear. I had never been afraid of flying or traveling in the past and I truly did not understand what was happening. I tried reading about how safe flying was and telling myself that this was irrational. I tried talking about it with my wife and talking through the fear. None of it worked. With less than a week before we were due to leave, I told my wife we were going to have to cancel. She suggested talking to Dr. Neimeyer after class, so I made an appointment and told Dr. Neimeyer my story. As we talked, we somehow ended up discussing my paper on the loss of my grandfather. With a little further discussion, I realized that writing that paper, and connecting to that experience of loss, had awakened something deep inside of me. My fear was not of me dying but of my boys not getting to know me if something happened on this trip. My solution was to write letters to each of them, talking about our relationship and my hopes and dreams for them, and placing them in a box next to my bed. This did not make the anxiety disappear but did make it manageable to where I could go on the trip and enjoy it. Now, every time I leave home on a trip without the children, I still write letters and keep them in a (now much larger) box.

This experience taught me a number of things about counseling: (1) Counseling needs to be directed at the level of meaning rather than only behavior or rational thought; (2) effective counseling does not have to be a long, complex procedure but can be as simple as a conversation; (3) insight is not enough—some type of meaningful action is necessary for change; (4) effective counseling does not necessarily remove the problem or pain but generates solutions that facilitate optimal functioning and engagement; and (5) details of a person's story that appear to an outsider to be unrelated to the current situation may, in fact, be crucial. I knew then that this was the type of approach to counseling that was needed in communication disorders.

As we discussed in the previous chapter, there are many barriers that prevent audiologists and speech-language pathologists from engaging in counseling, such as time pressure, lack of training, and misperceptions about what counseling involves and how it fits into EBP and the overall process of behavioral and technological treatment of communication disorders. Embedded in these barriers is a further problem that most speech-language pathologists and audiologists have with regard to engaging clients in counseling, and that is that they lack a systematic approach and struggle to facilitate the types of conversations that will help clients generate solutions to problems. What we have learned in our own experience as counselors and our dozen years of experience teaching counseling to speech-language pathology and audiology graduate students is that, in order for clinicians to actually engage in counseling, they need: (1) a basic theoretical framework to organize and guide the way they conceptualize their clients' problems, and (2) specific ways to engage clients in counseling conversations. With these two tools, clinicians can engage in counseling any clients in any context.

A Definitional Beginning

Just within the discipline of communication sciences and disorders, the term "counseling" is used to mean many different things. For example, audiologists frequently refer to the information-giving that they do following the dispensing of a hearing aid (or other assistive device) as "counseling." Similarly, speech-language pathologists will often refer to sessions in which they work with the parents of children who are in speech therapy as "parent counseling sessions." For others, the term "counseling" refers to a vague notion that they are supposed to talk to clients about their emotional reactions to their communication problems. Still others relate "counseling" to the course they had in their undergraduate or graduate program that presented a range of different psychotherapy approaches—none of which they learned enough about to actually try to use.

A number of authors have attempted to define "counseling" for the communication disorders field (e.g., Crowe, 1997; Flasher & Fogle, 2004; Luterman, 2008; Rollin, 2000; Shames, 2006), with the consensus being that, for speech-language pathologists and audiologists, counseling is a process by which clinicians help individuals and/or families manage, adjust to, and cope with communication and swallowing disorders. For the purposes of this text, we would also add "and the treatments for those disorders" to the above definition. Although this may at first appear strange, counseling in speech-language pathology and audiology often has as much to do with helping clients adjust to the treatments that they have received as it is about adjusting to the disorder itself (a lot more on this, later).

In the speech-language pathology and audiology literature, counseling is differentiated from psychotherapy primarily on the basis of the client population and related goals. For example, Crowe (1997), Rollin (2000), and Shames (2006) all agree that, despite using often similar or even identical approaches, the role of psychotherapy is to treat individuals who need to make personality changes due to psychological abnormalities, whereas the role of counseling is to treat essentially healthy individuals who require help adjusting to or coping with specific life events.

Levels of Counseling Intervention

Although the above definition of counseling as helping individuals and/or families manage, adjust to, and cope with communication and swallowing disorders and their treatments is helpful in a broad sense, it doesn't answer the question that we frequently get from both students and experienced clinicians alike: "How do I know if a particular client needs counseling?"

Our initial response to this question is rarely greeted with much enthusiasm by those who have asked, as the only reasonable answer is, "You don't!" We then have to elaborate further, explaining that if you are working from a conceptual framework in which you always consider the individual's personal story and the impact that his or her communication or swallowing disorder may have on that story, then you don't even need to ask the question; you are essentially always engaged in counseling, following the needs of the client as they unfold during your interactions, irrespective of what type of speech, language, swallowing, or audiologic treatments you are using.

Below, we have identified four broad levels of what might be termed "counseling intervention" that might help make this clearer for readers. It is important for readers to understand, however, that we would never "label" a client as "Level I" or "Level II" and so forth, with some implication of what counseling was to be done with them. In fact, it is assumed that clinicians will engage in Level I "counseling" with all clients, and then move in and out of other "levels" as might be needed on a session-by-session basis, always driven by the immediate and long-term needs of the client. Our purpose here is to make sure that readers understand that counseling is integrated into traditional speech, language, swallowing, and hearing treatments, and occurs with all clients, all the time, flowing from the needs of the client, not from the clinician's agenda.

Level I: Person-Centered Thinking

This is the most basic level and is the starting point with every client with whom clinicians interact. It is, essentially, the default way of thinking for the clinician, where the conceptual framework has become "second nature" and guides not only therapeutic decision-making but also the way that clients (and their families) are engaged in conversations. The client's communication or swallowing problems are conceptualized within the context of their broader "story," with attention focused at the level of meaning, not simply on observable behaviors and structures. It is not something that you include in a lesson plan or write a goal for; it is simply how you think and is fully integrated into the traditional practices and procedures that audiologists and speech-language pathologists are familiar with. All clients will benefit from this level of counseling intervention and, for some clients, this may be the only "counseling" that is needed. Additionally, included in this level is the "counseling" that occurs during information-giving sessions and any type of client or parent interviews.

The following description of an event experienced by one of our students provides a good example of this type of level I counseling:

The student described an encounter that she had with a patient in a nursing home. He was supposed to be evaluated by the speech-language pathologist early one morning but was agitated and non-compliant. The clinician spent some time trying to calm him down and get him to cooperate but with no success. While the clinician and nursing staff were discussing what to do with this gentleman, the student, who was accompanying the clinician, thought about what she had been learning in her counseling class. She quietly began by asking him to simply tell her about himself. She engaged him in a genuine conversation, each asking questions and telling stories, until he got around to telling her about an upsetting event that had happened with a family member the previous night. She responded by simply acknowledging that this must have been difficult for him but did not try to "fix" the situation. Following this conversation of no more than 10 minutes, the student reported that the man was fully compliant and easy to work with, and the assessment was completed within the time that had been scheduled.

In this example, the student was able to view this patient as a person with a story, rather than as simply a person to be assessed (and who was being non-compliant). Moreover, she was able to recognize that he needed to tell his story; he wanted to be listened to and was not interested in the agendas of the speech-language pathologist or the nursing staff. By engaging him in a conversation as a genuine, interested conversational partner, and by allowing him to tell his story, the student was eventually able to get to the meaning behind his behavior and, by acknowledging it, was able to help him move on, allowing the speech-language pathologist to then accomplish her goal of assessment.

Level II: Enhancing Conventional Therapies

This level builds on the first but is more deliberate because clients requiring this level of counseling intervention need help to create meaningful, long-term change in their lives. Clinicians might conceptualize this level as using counseling to enhance the "generalization" that clients (and clinicians) often struggle with in their behavioral interventions. For many clients, learning a new way to produce a certain sound, use their voice, control their fluency, or manage their hearing loss, is not a particularly difficult challenge. What is difficult, however, is learning to use those acquired behaviors in social, communicative situations outside of the therapy room. This is often when clinicians prescribe homework assignments and other techniques to enhance generalization. The problem, however, is not at the behavioral level (the clients can perform the behaviors) but at the level of meaning (there is something preventing them from performing the behaviors in those circumstances).

The following two clinical examples may be helpful to readers in understanding this "level" of counseling intervention:

Mark was a 22-year-old man who stuttered. He had been working on smoothing and controlling his stuttering for many years and was getting quite good at it. He was experiencing a period of relatively easy and consistent control over his disfluencies, a period that had been going for approximately 4 months, when we met after he had spent some time working at a school. Mark described to me an IEP meeting that he had been a part of and how he had been highly disfluent during the entire meeting. He told me that it had surprised him and he expressed frustration at his failure and had spent a lot of time analyzing why he had struggled. Rather than join Mark in his disappointment and analysis of where he had gone wrong behaviorally, I was excited. "I wonder if that tells you anything about how you are changing?" I said. Mark thought for a while; he didn't get it, so I helped a little. "I am trying to get you to think about how you might view this experience in an alternative way. So far, you have interpreted it as indicating that you need to practice your "technical" skills more. How might the fact that you were surprised by the stuttering tell you something about how you are changing in your thinking?" Again, Mark thought; and then he got it. "Okay, I think I know where you are going with this! Because I was surprised by the stuttering . . . it means that I wasn't expecting to stutter . . . which is a big change from what I would have expected before. Yeah, I see that. Hmm. That is kind of interesting!" We talked about this for some time. Mark struggled with the idea that he didn't expect to stutter—because a person who stutters always expects to stutter! This was a profound moment for Mark, as he began to realize that, at least in some ways, he was no longer thinking like a person who stutters. (See Chapter 9 for a more complete version of this conversation.)

Anna, a 5-year-old girl, had been working on correct production of several sounds for almost a year when we saw her at the University clinic. The first thing we noticed was that Anna produced few articulation errors during testing. Similarly, at various times when working with the clinician, Anna would produce her target sounds accurately. We also noticed that as soon as she came out of the therapy room and was interacting with her Mom, Anna reverted to her "typical" misarticulations. For a while, we tried a number of different "generalizing" tactics, having Anna producing the sounds correctly both in and out of the therapy room, with different clinicians, with Mom in the room, and setting homework assignments. Anna performed almost perfectly every time, but still continued to produce her typical speech patterns outside of the therapy room (and at times during therapy sessions as well).

Finally, we decided to ask Anna if she could help us out. We had her produce her "correct" speech and her "typical" speech. We then asked her which one she preferred and her answer told us everything we needed to know. She said, "This one," doing her typical speech. "Why?" we asked. Looking rather coy, the way only a 5-year-old girl can, she said, "Because Daddy likes it." Once we knew this, we were able to formulate an effective strategy that was meaningful to Anna (as opposed to the therapy that had been meaningful to us, the expert clinicians!). Of course, Anna was reluctant to give up a way of being that was clearly very important to her. It was also important for Anna's relationship with her father that he not simply tell her not to speak in that way, which could easily have been interpreted by Anna as rejection. Consequently, we decided to use some externalizing concepts (more on these in Chapters 8 and 11) and name the two speech roles that Anna was playing—"Little Anna" (for the misarticulated speech role) and "Big Anna" (for her accurate speech role). We started by asking Anna to perform speech tasks using each role, showing no preference for either. Anna's parents did the same at home, with particular emphasis on Dad asking for both roles during his interactions with Anna. Over the course of a few weeks, we (both clinicians and parents) gradually increased requests for "Big Anna" and reduced requests for "Little Anna." We also ensured that Anna's Dad asked for "Big Anna" during a number of father-daughter outings and games, helping Anna to specifically re-construct her self-image that had connected "Daddy's love and affection" with her "Little Anna" speech patterns. Within one semester, we were able to dismiss Anna from speech therapy.

Counseling at this level, then, helps clients to make sense of the behavioral changes that they are experiencing and to successfully integrate those new behaviors into their personal story. In the cases described above, Mark simply needed a conversation to help him to start to view the behavioral changes that he was making in more meaningful terms. For Anna, counseling took a more structured form but was still aimed at helping her to view the behavioral changes that she had learned as meaningful. In her case, the initial homework and generalizing activities did not work because they were not targeting the reason that she was not using the new behaviors. Once that reason was addressed, however, Anna was able to use her new behaviors successfully in all situations.

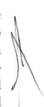

Level III: Changing Identities

This level of counseling is actually what most speech-language pathologists and audiologists think of when they think of counseling. At this level, counseling is a significant part of the therapeutic interaction. It may require time specifically allocated to counseling-type conversations (although speech and language targets may be practiced during these conversations) or may be integrated into whatever traditional speech, language, swallowing, or hearing treatment that is ongoing. Typically, only a few clients will require this level of counseling.

Another clinical example may be helpful to readers in understanding this "level" of counseling intervention:

Flora was a 76-year-old woman who had been having swallowing difficulties for some time, and when I first saw her in the nursing home, she had been on a pureed diet for almost two years. Although she had adjusted well to the diet within the confines of the nursing home, I learned from her family that she had not been out with them or to their home for a meal since the change in her diet, despite numerous invitations and encouragement. They did not know what to do and felt that their relationship with Flora was fading, as most of their family events revolved around meals.

After a few sessions with Flora in which we talked as much about her family as we did about her swallowing problems, I learned that she, also, felt less close to her family than before, and wanted very much to do something about it. I also learned, however, that she was extremely embarrassed and anxious about eating in front of anyone outside of the nursing home and could not imagine imposing her dietary needs on her family, or putting them though watching her eat pureed food. She resisted any suggestions that being family, they would not be bothered by her situation.

As Thanksgiving was only a few weeks away, I asked the family if we could work on getting Flora to have Thanksgiving dinner with them. They agreed and worked with me to arrange all the necessary accommodations that Flora would need. At first, Flora completely dismissed the idea. As we discussed it further, I asked Flora if she would be willing to try a series of "experiments" aimed at testing out some of her hypotheses about eating in public. By tentatively proposing these as experiments, it opened some space for Flora to think of them differently from regular events. She cautiously agreed and we discussed what I had in mind. We set up a series of experiments, starting with the least threatening and working towards Thanksgiving dinner with her family.

The first few experiments involved inviting various family members to the nursing home during meal times (Flora had previously refused to have them come during this time). We followed this with having Flora go to her daughter's home for a meal when the rest of the family was out. The final step was to have her go to the family's Thanksgiving dinner. To help Flora create meaningful cognitive change, each experiment was **preceded** *by having her make predictions about how things would* *turn out. We asked her to predict how she would feel (before, during, and after the meal), what things might go well and go badly (her fears), how the other people involved in the experiment would react, and what they might say.*

All of Flora's predictions were recorded in a notebook. Following the experiments, Flora and I discussed how it went, specifically reviewing each of her predictions. We found that many were not very accurate, particularly those related to her fears. We recorded these differences in her notebook as well, and I asked her to read through these notes frequently each day. At first it was uncomfortable for Flora to accept that her predictions were not accurate and she often attempted to explain why this experience might have just been an exception. As the series of experiments progressed, however, and many of her negative predictions continued to be invalidated, her resistance faded. Eventually, her predictions also began to change, with fewer predictions related to fear and embarrassment and more related to some positive experiences. By the time Thanksgiving arrived, Flora was willing to try eating with her whole family for the first time in over two years. The meal and her visit with the family went well and she continued to expand the number of meal-related events that she attended with her family.

In this example, no specific changes in the client's swallowing occurred. Yet, despite this, a significant improvement in quality of life occurred due to the speech-language pathologist's intervention. In this case, the experiments were not specifically related to traditional therapeutic activities. The process of experimenting and encouraging meaningful cognitive change, however, can be infused into many activities that speech-language pathologists and audiologists regularly engage their clients in, particularly those that place clients in new roles (e.g., using a hearing aid) or require them to practice newly acquired communication skills.

Level IV: Recognizing Limits

This level of counseling intervention occurs when clinicians recognize that a client's problems are beyond their capabilities or training to effectively deal with. This may mean that a client has deeper personality or mental health problems that, even if related to the communication disorder, are beyond the speech-language pathologist's or audiologist's training or scope of practice. It may also be, however, a client who has a particular problem (within the clinician's scope of practice) which a clinician feels she or he is not qualified to deal with or has some level of conflict of interest with (e.g., personal, religious, or financial). In these circumstances, clinicians refer either to other qualified speech-language pathologists or audiologists, or to physicians or clinicians in other fields such as psychology or social work.

Again, readers should note that categorizing counseling interventions into the four levels that we have discussed here is done as a matter of convenience to illustrate the varying types of interventions that can occur and the circumstances under which they might be useful. In practice, we would never "assess" a client and say, "this client will need Level III counseling intervention!" Working with real people, with real problems, is far too complex and fluid for such simple labeling. What we want to convey in this section is that all clients will benefit from some form of counseling, so clinicians do not need to ask questions about who needs counseling. Rather, clinicians need to develop a way of thinking that allows them to engage in all levels of counseling intervention as appropriate to the needs of a given case.

About This Book

Our goals for this book are to provide clinicians with: (1) a systematic approach with which to conceptualize counseling and their role as counselor and (2) a range of specific activities (a "toolbox") that clinicians can use to facilitate counseling conversations with clients who are working through any speech, language, swallowing, or hearing problem. The tools included in this book are not part of any prescribed process of counseling or psychotherapy— that is why we have avoided calling them "techniques"—and are not necessarily intended to have any therapeutic value in and of themselves. They are presented to aid clinicians in their creative engagements with their clients, fostering the types of therapeutic conversations that speech-language pathologists and audiologists often seem hesitant to engage in (i.e., conversations that go beyond taking about the communication problem and are reflective of the impact of the problem on the client's self image and quality of life). Clinicians are encouraged to experiment with different tools.

The book is organized into five parts; Part I: Getting Oriented; Part II: Theoretical Foundations; Part III: The Process of Counseling; Part IV: The Clinician's Toolbox; and Part V: Paying it Forward. Our intention is that Parts I to III of the book will be read in sequence, as concepts build from one chapter to the next. The chapters in Part IV are intended to be stand-alone chapters that can be read in any order as the need for different tools arises. The chapter and materials in Part V are intended to help instructors teach the constructivist counseling framework to students but may also provide clinicians with ideas for activities they might try to help sharpen their counseling skills.

Part I—Getting Oriented (3 chapters) consists of introductory chapters that describe issues related to counseling in speech-language pathology and audiology and how to integrate counseling into clinical practice. We introduce the idea that counseling for speech-language pathologists and audiologists is not necessarily the face-to-face verbal exchange that is traditionally thought of when we hear the word "counseling." Instead, audiologists and speech-language pathologists are *always* counseling and it is infused into all of our interactions with clients. For us, counseling is a way of *thinking* as much as it is a way of *doing*! We believe that Chapter 3, in particular, is of critical importance for clinicians and students to read, as it will help them grasp the foundational concept of "therapy as leadership" rather than service and help them to determine what aspects of a client's problem require more than simple "technical" intervention. With a leadership mentality, engaging clients in the process of counseling will be instinctive rather than foreign (as it seems to be for many clinicians).

Part II—Theoretical Foundations (5 chapters) establishes the theoretical groundwork for our approach to counseling. In this section, we review current approaches to counseling to help clinicians and students build an eclectic background from which to move forward. This general chapter is followed by specific chapters that introduce *constructivism* and *narrative therapy*, which are the foundations for the counseling framework to follow, and a chapter on the growing evidence for constructivist interpretations of communication disorders. The final chapter in this section (Chapter 8) describes in detail the specific framework that is the centerpiece of the book.

Part III—The Process of Counseling (5 chapters) expands on particular aspects of the constructivist counseling framework that was outlined in Chapter 8. The first two chapters in this section provide more detailed information on topics such as *listening, asking questions, using externalizing language, identifying iMoments, experimenting,* and *using outsider witnesses.* The final three chapters in this section provide three different clinical cases that illustrate specific aspects of the constructivist counseling process. In these case illustrations, we have tried to convey a sense of not only what actions occurred, but also the thought processes of the clinicians as they engaged with the clients. These cases provide readers with examples of how the framework might look in action—and remind readers that there are many different ways to engage clients and their families in effective counseling.

Part IV—Clinician's Toolbox (12 chapters) includes short chapters that each describe a tool that speech-language pathologists or audiologists might use to facilitate counseling interactions with their clients. Each of these short chapters is structured in an identical way to help readers build familiarity and confidence in using the "tool box." Each chapter includes: (1) indications of types of clients and/or situations with which the tool might be used, as well as any contraindications for use, (2) a list of materials needed, (3) a description of the tool, (4) a brief case example that illustrates the use of the tool, how it was implemented, what was learned from the client's responses, and how that information might be used to facilitate the counseling process, (5) concluding thoughts, and (6) "frequently asked questions" designed to answer questions clinicians might have about the tool and its use. These tools are drawn from a number of different theoretical traditions, but each has been chosen because it fits into the rationale and theoretical foundations of the constructivist counseling framework that we have presented in this book.

Part V—Paying it Forward (1 chapter) includes a chapter on how to approach teaching the constructivist counseling framework to speech-language pathology and audiology students. It also includes materials such as example activities, assignments, and grading rubrics that instructors might find useful as they prepare to teach counseling to students.

In summary, we have found counseling to be an essential part of our work with people who consult us with a great range of communication problems, and trust that the chapters that follow will convey something of the spirit and substance of an approach to this work that we have found immensely practical. So let's continue in this invitational mood and turn to the foundation for all of the specific tools to follow, namely, the stance of the therapist.

References

Crowe, T. A. (Ed.) (1997). *Applications of counseling in speech-language pathology and audiology.* Philadelphia, PA: Williams & Wilkins.

Flasher, L., & Fogle, P. (2004). *Counseling skills for the speech-language pathologist and audiologist.* Clifton Park, NY: Thomson-Delmar Learning.

Luterman, D. M. (2008). *Counseling persons with communication disorders and their families.* (5th ed.). Austin, TX: Pro-Ed, Inc.

Rollin, W. J. (2000). *Counseling individuals with communication disorders: Psychodynamic and family aspects* (2nd ed.). Boston, MA: Butterworth-Heinemann.

Shames, G. H. (2006). *Counseling the communicatively disabled and their families: A manual for clinicians.* Mahwah, NJ: Lawrence Erlbaum Associates.

3

THE LEADERSHIP OF THERAPY: HOW TO INTEGRATE COUNSELING INTO YOUR CLINICAL PRACTICE

One of the primary goals of this book is to help clinicians understand that *counseling* is something that is part of who they are and how they think, not merely something that they do! One way of thinking about this is to consider counseling as described in Chapter 2, where we described four levels of "counseling intervention." Most speech-language pathologists and audiologists typically think that they are "doing" counseling if they are engaged in Level III types of interventions. Our point, of course, is that Level I and II types of interventions are also "counseling" and, in fact, not only set the ground work for more formal counseling interactions (Level III) but also are relevant to more clients.

In this chapter, we look at the therapeutic interaction through a different lens: that of adaptive leadership. In health-care settings, speech-language pathologists and audiologists are often referred to as "service providers" and, consequently, are expected to "provide" "service" to the clients who come to see them. This model implies a passive, broken client who comes to the expert clinician to be fixed, hardly a model that encourages the type of counseling that we are advocating in this book. What if, instead of viewing what we do as clinicians as providing a "service," we were to view what we do as "leadership?"

Complex Adaptive Systems

A "complex adaptive system" may be defined as "a collection of individual agents with freedom to act in ways that are not always totally predictable, and whose actions are interconnected so that the action of one part changes the context for other agents" (Wilson, Holt, & Greenhalgh, 2001; p. 685). The concept of complex adaptive systems has typically been used to describe organizations, but, recently, some authors have suggested that it may also apply to individuals in that individuals adapt both physically and psychologically as they interact with their changing environment (Bailey, et al., 2012; Thygeson, Morrissey, & Ulstad, 2010). This new perspective, therefore, may help us to understand why we often fail when treating the complex "human system" as a simple "cause-and-effect" system.

A consequence of this complex adaptive system view of the individual is that we can no longer apply the traditional (linear) medical model to illness and disability. The medical model likens the human body to a machine and the malfunctioning of that "machine" to a breakdown of its component parts, considering each part in isolation. By definition, then, such a linear model necessitates breaking down clinical intervention into smaller units to focus on treating the individual components. Complexity science, on the other hand, suggests that illness and health result from complex, dynamic, and unique interactions between different components of the overall system. The clinical implication of this view, therefore, is that effective clinical decision making will require a holistic approach that understands that malfunctioning components are part of an overall dynamic system that is impacted by that malfunction.

In the business world, interventions designed to address problems within complex adaptive systems such as large organizations and institutions have been developed through what has been termed *adaptive leadership* (e.g., Heifetz, Grashow, & Linsky, 2009; Heifetz & Laurie, 1997; Heifetz & Linsky, 2002). These same principles of adaptive leadership have been suggested as a useful framework for clinical encounters (e.g., Bailey et al., 2012; DiLollo, 2010; Thygeson et al., 2010). The remainder of this chapter outlines the basic tenets of adaptive leadership, and how it might be useful in guiding clinical decision-making for speech-language pathologists and audiologists.

Adaptive Leadership

Typically, when we mention the word "leadership," people think of someone in a position of authority or power—a CEO, a principal, a senator. The stance taken by proponents of adaptive leadership (e.g., Heifetz et al., 2009; Heifetz & Laurie, 1997; Heifetz & Linsky, 2002), however, is that "leadership is an activity, not a position" (Cohen & Tedesco, 2009, p. 5). They see authority, power, and influence as useful *tools* but emphasize that these tools "do not define leadership" (Heifetz et al., 2009, p. 24). In this view, then, authority relationships are seen as "power entrusted for service" (p. 24), suggesting that individuals attain positions of authority with the expectation that they will provide some kind of *service* to those under them. In contrast, Heifetz and his colleagues (2009) describe *adaptive leadership* as "the practice of mobilizing people to tackle tough challenges and thrive" (p. 14).

At the core of the concept of adaptive leadership lies the distinction between two broad categories of challenges that people face: *technical* and *adaptive* challenges. *Technical challenges* are situations where both the problem and the solution can be clearly defined by an "expert" and, as such, are best addressed by an expert in a position of authority. *Adaptive challenges*, on the other hand, have no known solution, and the skills and answers require changes in behaviors and ways of thinking (Heifetz & Laurie, 1997; Heifetz & Linsky, 2002). Adaptive challenges, therefore, must be addressed by the "stakeholders"—that is, the individuals or group who must make the changes to their thinking and behavior. O'Malley (2009) viscerally described the differences between technical and adaptive challenges this way: "Technical problems live in people's heads and logic systems. They are susceptible to facts and authoritative expertise. Adaptive challenges live in people's hearts and stomachs. They are about values, loyalties, and beliefs. Progress on them requires the people with the problem to do the work, and the work involves refashioning those deeply held beliefs" (p. 9).

Many problems faced by individuals and organizations contain elements of *both* technical and adaptive challenges. According to Heifetz et al. (2009), one of the most common leadership mistakes is attempting to address adaptive challenges with technical solutions. Similarly, addressing technical challenges with adaptive interventions would clearly be a waste of time and energy, with little chance of success. Consequently, it is important to distinguish between these two types of challenges in order to design the most appropriate interventions.

Four Competencies for Engaging in Adaptive Work

The Kansas Leadership Center has taken the work of Heifetz and colleagues and described a set of 'competencies" (Table 3–1) aimed at helping people engage in adaptive leadership (McBride, 2011).

Diagnose the Situation

This is where time is taken to distinguish between technical and adaptive elements of the problem and to consider multiple interpretations of the situation. Of importance here is that default interpretations are not simply accepted but are questioned and challenged, as, in most cases, default interpretations tend to be very technical in nature. A further aspect of this competency is related to what

Table 3–1. Four Competencies for Engaging In Adaptive Work

1. Diagnose the situation	Distinguish the technical and adaptive elements
	Test multiple interpretations
	Push against default interpretations—which tend to be technical
	Read temperature in the system
2. Manage self	Identify your capabilities, vulnerabilities, and triggers
	Distinguish self from role
	Understand the role you play in the system
	Choose among competing values
	Increase tolerance for uncertainty, ambiguity, and conflict
3. Intervene skillfully	Capture attention
	Raise or lower the heat
	Give the work back
	Create conditions for collaboration
	Act experimentally: Experiment beyond your comfort zone (i.e., do what is needed, not what is comfortable)
4. Energize others	Engage unusual voices
	Speak from the heart
	Speak to the loss
	Empowerment
	Start where they are, not where you are

Heifetz and Laurie (1997) term "the heat" or temperature of the system. This is referring to disequilibrium in the system and how much discomfort it produces. For example, if a problem is not producing much discomfort, there is little motivation for stakeholders to make significant change. Similarly, if too much discomfort is produced by a problem, stakeholders may become immobilized or be too distracted to accomplish meaningful change. Consequently, understanding the "temperature" of the system is important when planning any type of adaptive intervention.

Manage Self

In order to engage in adaptive leadership, individuals need to be aware of their own role in the process. This entails considering your own capabilities and vulnerabilities and how they might affect your role in the process. Triggers are things that may come up during the leadership process that might distract you because of some personal issues. For example, if you react defensively to being challenged, this might be a trigger for you and may impede progress. Similarly, it is important for leaders to see themselves as separate from their role, thus enabling them to exclude their own issues and triggers from the process. There are often competing values in any situation and, as a leader, it is important to be able to recognize these and choose among them to facilitate positive change. Finally, when faced with a problem situation, many individuals want things to change quickly. Adaptive challenges seldom have "quick fixes" and typically require patience and tolerance of uncertainty, ambiguity, and conflict to allow the process to evolve.

Intervene Skillfully

This competency focuses on what the leader can do to intervene in the situation. In adaptive leadership, intervention is not about "solving" the problem. Rather, it is about giving the work back to the stakeholders (as they are the only ones who can make the adaptive changes that will be needed) and motivating them to do the hard work that is needed for change to occur. As such, leaders may play a role in raising or lowering the "heat" (see Competency #1) as needed to facilitate a "productive zone of disequilibrium" (Heifetz & Laurie, 1997). Typically, adaptive leaders will engage stakeholders in "experiments" that test out new behaviors and new ways of thinking. It is important for experimentation to be outside of "comfort-zones" so that it moves behavior and/or thinking to new places.

Energize Others

This competency focuses on motivating stakeholders to engage in, and persist with, the adaptive work needed to address the problem. Adaptive leaders need to be genuine and speak from the heart. This means not being afraid of the "difficult" conversations that frequently occur when helping people to change adaptively. Similarly, adaptive work always leads to loss—loss of "the way things have always been done," loss of status, loss of comfort, and so forth—and leaders must recognize stakeholders' loss and be willing to address it. It is also important for adaptive leaders to recognize that stakeholders may not have the same perspective on the problem as they do. Given this, it is useful for leaders to engage "unusual voices"—people who may not be part of the main body of stakeholders—to get different perspectives and interpretations of the problem and situation. Finally, leaders must recognize that the process needs to start at the point of the stakeholders' understanding of the problem, not the leaders'.

Therapy and Counseling as an Act of Leadership

Consider the following quote: "To practice adaptive leadership, you have to help people navigate through a period of disturbance as they sift through what is essential and what is expendable, and as they experiment with solutions to the adaptive challenges at hand" (Heifetz, Grashow, & Linsky, 2009, p. 28). This quote neatly summarizes the task at hand for clinicians when confronted with a client with a communication problem. Typically, clients come to us with communication problems that are part technical and part adaptive. Our role is to help them navigate though "a period of disturbance" (the speech, language, or hearing treatment causes the "disturbance" as it threatens to change the way the individual has functioned in the past) and to decide what and how much they are willing to change. We often do this by helping clients "experiment" with different ways of behaving and thinking. Lets take a look at a clinical example:

> *Tori is a 16-year-old girl who is being seen for a voice disorder due to vocal nodules. Tori is a very extraverted, talkative girl who is a cheerleader at school and tends to press hard with her voice in almost all situations. The **technical** aspect of Tori's problem is the voice disorder and learning the behavioral changes needed for remediation; the **adaptive** aspect involves the associated lifestyle and self-image changes that Tori will need to adopt for long-term behavioral change to occur. The "period of disturbance" would be the speech therapy: typically, vocal rest, use of a less intense, breathy voice, and improved vocal hygiene. Tori will need to decide what changes she is willing to make, what parts of her self (our vocal characteristics form a big part of our self-image) she is willing to give up (the loss associated with adaptive change) to achieve her voice goals. The role of the therapist is to help Tori **experiment** with different roles that may achieve some or all of her goals. If the therapist simply tries to implement a technical solution (e.g., teaches Tori the new voice she is to use and sets up a behavioral monitoring schedule), chances are that Tori will change her behaviors temporarily but will go back to her usual ways soon after dismissal from therapy.*

By conceptualizing therapy as an act of *adaptive leadership*, it is possible to see how our role is more than simple (technical) behavior change and how we need to be thinking in terms of facilitating *adaptive change* in addition to the behavior change—and that is exactly the role that counseling plays in the therapeutic process.

Four Competencies for Engaging in Adaptive Work—Revisited

As a way of helping clinicians map concepts from adaptive leadership onto the therapeutic process, let us revisit the four competencies described earlier but frame them in terms of clinical interactions typically seen by speech-language pathologists (SLPs) and audiologists.

Diagnose the Situation

Almost always, communication problems present with BOTH technical and adaptive challenges. It is important for clinicians to identify both of these types of challenges if they are to facilitate long-term, meaningful change for their clients. Typically, technical challenges are related to the specific communication problem and can be assessed and treated via the traditional behavioral and technological methods used by speech-language pathologists and audiologists. Adaptive challenges, however, are related to changes that are needed in less tangible areas such as beliefs, self-image, and lifestyle; changes that are critical for the long-term adoption of the technical behavioral/technological solutions. This is where counseling and person-centered care are of vital importance. In speech-language pathology and audiology, default interpretations relate primarily to the linear, medical model that conceptualizes illness as a breakdown in components, and treatment as repairing those malfunctioning components (a highly technical approach). It is important for speech-language pathologists and audiologists to question and challenge these default interpretations and extend their understanding of communication disorders in more adaptive ways. Finally, clinicians working with clients with communication problems will need to read the temperature of the system. In many cases, the communication problem may have become too easy for the client to live with, making the prospect of engaging in adaptive work quite unappealing (i.e., the heat is too low for productive disequilibrium). Conversely, for some clients, the communication problem might be so overwhelming that they simply cannot deal with it. An example of this might be seen with persons who stutter—for some persons who stutter (PWS) who are good at avoiding and ignoring their stuttering, it is easier to live with the problem than to put forth the effort and sacrifice to monitor and modify their speech. In such cases, the clinician might work with the client to produce more open stuttering, thus raising the "heat" of the system; for others, their fear of stuttering is so overwhelming that they cannot engage in effective therapeutic activities. Thus, desensitization activities might be one way that the clinician regulates the "temperature" of the system so that it is at a more manageable level that will allow the client to engage in the process of change.

Manage Self

In order to engage in adaptive leadership, clinicians need to be aware of their own role in the process. This can be somewhat complicated for clinicians as we essentially play two roles, one as the technical "expert" in a position of authority, and one as an adaptive leader, recognizing (and valuing) the knowledge, capabilities and resources of clients and their ability to change. Recognizing this dual role (rather than simply staying with the default, technical role) and identifying technical and adaptive aspects of the problem can help clinicians deal with this issue.

In the clinical setting, triggers are often related to client characteristics such as looks, personality, mannerisms, dress, or accent. Such things can trigger reactions in clinicians that can impede the therapeutic process. Clinicians should be aware of their triggers and actively work against their influence.

There are often competing values in clinical environments (e.g., values of the client; the family; other clinicians; employers/supervisors; the facility; the health care or educational system) and clinicians must recognize these and choose among them to facilitate positive change. Many clinicians want therapy to progress quickly and, although the technical aspects of the therapeutic process may sometimes progress rapidly, adaptive challenges typically require patience and tolerance of uncertainty, ambiguity, and conflict to allow the process to evolve.

Intervene Skillfully

Working adaptively in clinical situations means that the interventions that you try are not aimed at "solving" the problem but are designed to give the work back to the client (the stakeholder), as he or she is the only one who can make the changes in beliefs, thinking, self-image, or lifestyle that are needed. The clinician's role is to motivate clients to do the hard work that is needed for change to occur. In this sense, clinicians play a role in manipulating the "heat" as needed to facilitate the productive zone of disequilibrium referred to earlier. One of the most powerful tools available to clinicians to facilitate adaptive work is to engage clients in "experiments" that test out not only new communication behaviors but also new ways of thinking and feeling. (In subsequent chapters, there will be a lot more about experimenting as it is a hallmark of constructivist approaches to counseling).

Energize Others *decide → loss*

Many authors have discussed the need for clinicians to be genuine, empathic, and charismatic (e.g., Manning, 2010; Van Riper, 1975). Not surprisingly, these traits are also important in facilitating adaptive work with clients—the speaking from the heart referred to previously. Clinically speaking, the technical work that we do with clients is not typically very painful, either physically or emotionally. When faced with adaptive work, however, things don't always go as smoothly, often resulting in clients being labeled "non-compliant" or simply dropping out of therapy. Clinicians need to recognize the influence of adaptive challenges and be ready to engage clients in those "difficult" conversations that address the discomfort and potential loss of adaptive work. Loss in the therapeutic environment can take the form of loss of self-image (even a self-image built on disorder can be difficult to relinquish), loss of control, loss of dreams and expectations, loss of feeling "normal" or complete, and many others. Finally, it is important for clinicians to recognize that clients may not have the same perspective on the problem as they do. Therefore, it is necessary to always get the clients' perspective on their problem (i.e., they are they expert on their problem) and to also engage those "unusual voices"—friends, family, co-workers, and even other clients and clinicians—to get different perspectives and interpretations of the problem and situation.

Conclusion

Two of the most common questions we are asked by both speech-language pathologists and audiologists about counseling are, "When do I do counseling?" and "How do I know what aspects of my client's problem require counseling?" The purpose of this chapter was: (1) to help clinicians view their role in therapy as one of *adaptive leadership* rather than service, thereby obviating the need to ask the question "when do I do counseling?" because an adaptive leader approaches problems in a way that automatically has the clinician take a counseling perspective (so, in essence, the clinician is always counseling); and (2) to help clinicians distinguish between the *technical* and *adaptive* aspects of clinical problems, thus enabling them to more clearly define those aspects of clients' problems that require more behavioral or technological (technical) approaches and those that require a more counseling-based (adaptive) approach. With that distinction in mind, we are now ready to explore the wide world of counseling, with special focus on its relevance for the field of communication disorders.

References

Bailey, D. E., Docherty, S. L., Adams, J. A., Carthron, D. L., Corazzini, K., Day, J. R., . . . Anderson, R. A. (2012). Studying the clinical encounter with the Adaptive Leadership framework. *Journal of Healthcare Leadership, 4*, 83–91.

Cohen, P. A., & Tedesco, L. A. (2009). Willing, ready, and able? How we must exercise leadership for needed change in dental education. *Journal of Dental Education, 73*, 3–11.

DiLollo, A. (2010). Constructivism and adaptive leadership: Framing an approach for SLPs and audiologists to overcome barriers to counseling. In R. J. Fourie (Ed.), *Therapeutic Processes for Communication Disorders* (Chapter 11, pp. 139–152). London, UK: Psychology Press.

Heifetz, R. A., Grashow, A., & Linsky, M. (2009). *The practice of adaptive leadership.* Boston, MA: Harvard Business Press.

Heifetz, R. A., & Laurie, D. L. (1997). The work of leadership. *Harvard Business Review, 75*, 124–134.

Heifetz, R. A., & Linsky, M. (2002). *Leadership on the line.* Boston, MA: Harvard Business Press.

Manning, W. H. (2010). *Clinical decision making in fluency disorders* (3rd ed.). Clifton Park, NY: Delmar, Cengage Learning.

McBride, J. F. (2011). *Civic leadership coaching: A handbook for coaches and leadership program developers.* Wichita, KS: The Kansas Leadership Center.

O'Malley, E. (2009). The competencies for civic leadership. *The Journal of Kansas Civic Leadership Development, 1,* 7-15.

Thygeson, M., Morrissey, L., & Ulstad, V. (2010). Adaptive leadership and the practice of medicine: A complexity-based approach to reframing the doctor-patient relationship. *Journal of Evaluation in Clinical Practice, 16,* 1009-1015.

Van Riper, C. (1975). The stutterer's clinician. In J. Eisenson (Ed.), *Stuttering, a second symposium* (pp. 453-492). New York, NY: Harper & Row.

Wilson, T., Holt, T., & Greenhalgh, T. (2001). Complexity science: Complexity and clinical care. *British Medical Journal, 323,* 685-688.

Part II

THEORETICAL FOUNDATIONS

The five chapters in Part II are designed to provide readers with background knowledge in general psychotherapy as well as the foundational psychotherapy traditions—personal construct psychology and narrative therapy—that form the foundation of the constructivist counseling framework that is presented at the end of the section.

4

OVERVIEW OF APPROACHES TO COUNSELING

In an important sense, the field of speech and language pathology evolved from the discipline of counseling and psychotherapy;[1] just as the latter profession was in part an outgrowth of philosophy. In this brief chapter, we offer a guided tour of some of the major traditions of counseling as they are practiced by psychologists and other helping professionals, and briefly consider their implications for the sort of counseling that is helpful in working with people with communication disorders. But lest the reader imagine that this

---

[1] In this chapter we use the terms counseling and psychotherapy roughly interchangeably, as both are concerned with the predominantly verbal exchange between a professional and a client, the goal of which is to assess, clarify, and surmount problems in living so that the client might live with less distress and greater satisfaction. Doing so at this point in the book also recognizes the relevance of historical "psychotherapy" theories for counseling in communication disorders. However, in the latter field, psychotherapy implies more of a "doctor–patient" style of relationship, in which psychological disorders are formally diagnosed and treated, whereas counseling implies a more humanistic and growth-promoting interaction in which clients are supported or coached in pursuing desired changes. For this reason we will focus on "counseling" in subsequent chapters.

is a comprehensive survey, it is worth noting that some observers have identified as many as 400 "name brands" of psychotherapy! This being the case, our overview is highly selective and focuses on major orientations or traditions, each of which encompasses many variations.[2] We start more or less at the beginning, with the pioneering work of Sigmund Freud.

Freud and Psychoanalysis

All too often, contemporary students and even professors of psychology roll their eyes at the mention of Sigmund Freud (1856–1939), identifying him with an emphasis on the role of hidden sexual motivation in driving human activity as revealed in dreams, slips of the tongue, and the dynamics of close relationships, especially with one's parents. But while these themes do characterize Freud's thought, they also caricature it, minimizing or misunderstanding his more enduring contributions to the conceptualization of human suffering and contemporary attempts to mitigate it in the context of psychotherapy. Here we, like most practicing psychoanalysts, will focus on his broader assumptions about people's psychological processes, and how a therapist helps clients develop greater awareness and agency about how they are living so that change becomes possible (Freud, 1940).

A fundamental assumption of Freud's was that much of mental life was *unconscious*, meaning that it occurred outside awareness, making reflection upon and discussion of it difficult under normal circumstances. This view accords well with contemporary research in cognitive neuroscience, which acknowledges that most human perceptions, actions, and beliefs are highly "automated," occurring more or less on their own, without our conscious deliberation (Westen, 1998). For example, if we were asked exactly how we maintain our balance on a bicycle or what facial muscles

---

[2] Readers interested in getting more deeply acquainted with the lively field of psychotherapy and counseling are encouraged to consult recent texts by Messer and Gurman (2011) and Sommers-Flanagan and Sommers-Flanagan (2012).

we watched to tell a true smile from a false one, most of us would be hard pressed to say. These and countless other particulars simply fall outside our awareness, yet continue to function in a way that shapes our experience and actions. Freud's emphasis was on how such unconscious patterns play out across the course of our lives, and especially in our close relationships, when we "transfer" half-forgotten models of relating learned with earlier figures into current situations. When this happens—as when a young man who was frequently belittled as a boy by his father automatically approaches later authority figures with a chip on his shoulder—we are prone to re-enact maladaptive cycles of interaction without realizing why. Psychoanalysis helps take such patterns out of "automatic" and make them more open to review and revision.

A second key theme in psychoanalytic perspectives is the assumption that much of mental life is characterized by *conflict*, that is by a sense of anxiety that arises from the way we relate to experiences and to ourselves. One classic expression of this is when we desire one thing (such as a dating relationship with an attractive partner), but block ourselves from pursuing it by an act of internal self-criticism or prohibition (such as telling ourselves that we don't deserve such attention or love, or that physical intimacy would be wrong because of religious beliefs about sex). These sorts of clashes between the desiring part of our self (the *id*) and the moralistic or evaluative part (the *superego*) can either generate a reasonable compromise (such as approaching and getting to know the other, to see what might develop) by drawing on our rational skills (the *ego*), or lead to considerable inner conflict. In the latter case, we might resort to all manner of *defensive maneuvers* to mitigate our distress, such as rationalizing that we really weren't that attracted to the other to begin with, or projecting our self-criticism on the other, and being overly vigilant for subtle signs of rejection.

As a form of treatment, psychoanalysis helps people recognize when they are engaging in unconscious, automatic, or defensive behaviors, and honestly take stock of their real needs and wishes. This is done in an environment in which the client speaks freely about his or her experience with minimal interference by the analyst, whose main role is to help the client acknowledge troubling feelings and decisions honestly, and develop insight about how these problematic patterns arose to begin with. Armed with greater awareness in a non-evaluative treatment relationship with a concerned and interested professional, the client is then in a better position to challenge and change unsatisfying patterns, and reach toward a more courageous and fulfilling way of living.

How might a psychoanalytic orientation inform counseling for communication disorders? In keeping with the central roles of anxiety, conflict, and defense, a psychoanalytic orientation would suggest that the speech therapist or audiologist let the client talk freely, and listen for how he or she manages anxiety—say, the nervousness of producing speech sounds in a new (correct) way in a social situation, or of participating in a noisy party as someone with partial hearing loss. Helping clients acknowledge their fears honestly and develop rational strategies for addressing them—rather than making excuses for their avoidance or projecting blame onto others—could then follow. Likewise, tuning an analytic ear to conflicts within the client—as when one part wants to be a fuller participant in the social world while another part stands back and harshly criticizes the client's best efforts—can be important, regardless of the technical intervention to assist with communication that the clinician is pursuing. Not uncommonly, clients may also fall into old, unconscious patterns that perpetuate problems, such as passively going along with ideas suggested by others to keep from "making waves," a tendency that the clinician might note that the client also engages in during therapy. Observing this in a non-critical way ("I wonder if you sometimes agree with me just to avoid an argument, when you really think differently about the issue. Is this something you notice yourself doing with other people, too?") can help the client be more self-aware of such patterns in communication situations, and step away from habitual ways that he or she unintentionally perpetuates unsatisfying interactions.

Rogers and Humanistic Therapy

Carl Rogers (1902–1987) was among the early contributors to humanistic psychology, a tradition that values human dignity and individuality, and sees counseling as less a matter of curing psychopathology than as a context for fostering personal growth. This is not to say that people do not suffer from significant distress and unhappiness, but rather that in an appropriate therapeutic environment they can move toward greater self-compassion and self-understanding, and ultimately greater authenticity in their lives with others. From this perspective, the role of the counselor is to construct with the client just this sort of growth-enhancing environment.

At the core of Roger's person-centered approach is the responsive but nondirective stance of the therapist, as reflected in his or her *accurate empathy* (really hearing and reflecting the client's concerns or feelings), *genuineness* (cultivating a person-to-person relationship with the client, rather than a distancing professional one), and *unconditional positive regard* (accepting and appreciating the fundamental humanity of the client, even when the counselor disagrees with his or her behavior) (Rogers, 1961). Typically this stance is conveyed in the counselor's deeply reflective listening to the client, more than by any direct statement to the client about his or her attitudes or recommendations. For example, if a client who experiences difficulty swallowing some weeks after a mild stroke were to say, "I don't know. . . . I just don't enjoy things like I used to, and I feel self-conscious at mealtimes with my family," the counselor might say, "It sounds sort of depressing to have to work on something like eating that you once took for granted, especially when you feel others looking at you differently." Such a response acknowledges the client's implied feelings, especially in a social setting now made awkward by the swallowing disorder, and sets the stage for joint problem solving. Or in working with a child who is being bullied about his articulation errors, the clinician might respond in an age- appropriate way by saying, "It must really make you mad when kids pick on you just because you talk different." These sorts of empathic reflections obviously take little time in the session, and can earn the client's trust and cooperation with other aspects of the therapy. This was well illustrated by the vignette of the student whose active listening to the angry nursing home resident in Chapter 2 allowed them to move past an initial impasse and cooperate fully on the clinical assessment that the resident had been resisting.

At another level, the counselor's positive regard can help counter what Rogers termed *conditions of worth* imposed on the client throughout life—the sense that he or she "didn't measure up" in some fashion, or that the problem or handicap represents a source of shame. Listening intently and without impatience as a disfluent client describes his or her difficulty, and accepting the associated feelings as understandable, can build a working alliance that can energize treatment, and convey genuine respect for the person with the problem. This sort of counseling relationship can itself be healing and reduce the client's anxiety and self-consciousness, promoting greater client receptivity and perseverance in other aspects of the treatment. In this book, techniques that involve inviting *Thick Descriptions* of relevant experiences (Chapters 8 & 9) and listening for *Innovative Moments* that augur for change (Chapters 8 & 10) are partly inspired by the appreciative, responsive stance of humanistic counseling, and reinforce the client's role as an active participant in making therapy work.

Wolpe and Behavior Therapy

Joseph Wolpe (1915–1997) was a pioneering figure in behavior therapy, introducing *systematic desensitization* as a popular technique for dealing with anxiety-producing situations of all kinds, ranging from fear of flying to social phobia (Wolpe, 1958). Hallmarks of behavioral approaches include the systematic, practical focus on careful assessment, and step-by-step methods for learning new skills to manage stressful circumstances or develop new competencies. Thus, in this technique, the behavior therapist first elicits a comprehensive picture of situations that trigger the client's distress in a given domain, working with him or her to organize them into a *fear hierarchy* that builds from mild discomfort to paralyzing dread. The clinician then coaches the client on various breathing techniques or progressive muscle relaxation, in order to induce an emotional state that is incompatible with anxiety. As the client becomes more practiced at producing this state of relaxed alertness, he or she is asked to do so while conjuring an image of the first and lowest item on the fear hierarchy. When the client can do this while managing not to become emotionally aroused, the clinician introduces the next higher situation on the hierarchy, and therapy continues until the client can master each of the initially anxious situations without incapacitating fear or avoidance. The same principles can inform therapeutic *homework* or "field trials" in which the client tries approaching a series of increasingly anxiety-arousing circumstances while maintaining a reasonable level of relaxation. Nowadays biofeedback or neurofeedback sometimes is added to this basic regimen to help clients monitor their anxiety levels while in the presence of the real or imagined stressor. Further extensions of a behavior therapy approach entail careful analysis of the contexts in which maladaptive responses occur in order to look for factors that can *reinforce* suboptimal coping, such as the reduction in stress that follows postponing rather than engaging an important but difficult task. The behavior therapist then collaborates with the client to find positive reinforcers (praise, tangible rewards) for good efforts, and administers these (or coaches the client to do so) as treatment progresses until the new and adaptive behavior is well established.

Obviously, many aspects of behavior therapy inform interventions in the communication disorders field, particularly the prompting, shaping, and reinforcing of speech and language production in the context of speech therapy. What is sometimes missed is that many of these same behavioral principles have a role in "counseling" dimensions of such work, as when a fear hierarchy of challenging social situations can be constructed that clients can be guided to engage in once they acquire skills in emotion regulation and relaxation techniques. Subsequent discussions of methods such as *Experimenting with Experience* (Chapter 21) and *Mindfulness* (Chapter 25) are coherent with many of the precepts of behavior therapy, even though they also draw on other approaches, and *Therapeutic Documents* (Chapter 24) can serve as a powerful reinforcement of client progress. Thus, counseling can be considered a natural outgrowth of more technical interventions (e.g., shaping articulation or fitting an assistive device), rather than something calling for an altogether different way of working.

Aaron Beck and Cognitive Therapy

As a psychiatrist working extensively with depressed and anxious patients, Aaron Beck (born 1921) was struck by the relevance of their conscious thoughts and preoccupations to the development and maintenance of their symptoms (Beck, 1976). Thus, depressed patients tended to anticipate and interpret experiences in terms of a *cognitive triad* that focused on *self* as a failure or as unlovable, the *world* as remote or rejecting, and the *future* as bleak or devoid of fulfillment. In contrast, anxious patients tended to think of the *self* as weak or vulnerable, the *world* as dangerous or unreliable, and the *future* as foreboding or uncertain. As a result, when encountering an ambiguous social situation, the former would tend to fixate on the likelihood of being defeated or rejected, whereas the latter would tend to read situations as threatening or overwhelming. Both patterns could become self-fulfilling prophecies, as the thoughts and associated emotions could lead to behaviors (such as overdependence on others or withdrawal) that could compound the problem.

Borrowing from behavior therapy perspectives with which it often allies, cognitive therapy concentrates on the careful delineation and treatment of problems in the contexts in which they occur. This translates into an effort at tracing, critiquing, and disputing self-defeating patterns of thinking by testing them out in real life situations or seeking more rational alternatives. For example, a cognitive therapist would be alert to certain *cognitive errors* such as *mind-reading* (presuming to know the intentions or reactions of others without checking them out), *all-or-nothing thinking* (thinking in extreme terms such as success vs. failure, with no shades of gray between), or *fortune telling* (anticipating negative outcomes with insufficient evidence to warrant this). Importantly, the therapist would strive to motivate the clients to monitor their thinking in problem situations not only within sessions, but also between them, recognizing the fundamental role of between session homework in this approach (Neimeyer, Kazantzis, Kassler, Baker, & Fletcher, 2008). Often this takes the form of having clients write about their thinking when they become aware of a strong negative emotion, analyzing circular or maladaptive patterns, and substituting more adaptive ones.

The focus on anticipatory anxiety and self-evaluation that characterizes cognitive approaches is relevant to many communication disorders, and the practical focus on self-observation and experimentation can easily inform counseling for these conditions. For example, heightened levels of cognitive anxiety have been found in people consulting for hearing evaluations, as discussed in Chapter 7, suggesting the importance of attending to their anticipation of difficulties in communication situations, and adaptive or less adaptive ways of dealing with these. Similarly, global and extreme forms of self-evaluation could characterize clients' engagement in speech modification in real-world settings, leading to harsh self-criticism for perceived failures, when in fact they may have been substantially, if not perfectly, successful in their efforts. A focus on how people think about themselves and their problems characterizes many of the techniques presented in Part IV, including the *Autobiography of the Problem* (Chapter 15), *Dear John Letter* (Chapter 18), and the *Self-Characterization* (Chapter 20).

Conclusion

As noted in Chapter 1, the defining ASHA documents for the field of communication disorders recognizes that counseling is an inherent and appropriate part of the job description of speech-language therapists and audiologists. Despite this, many practitioners have been reluctant to borrow from the various traditions of psychotherapy, partly out of the concern that this would place them on a slippery slope toward treating the "psychological problems" of their clients, rather than focusing on remediating their communication difficulties. Our view in this chapter and throughout the book is that this is in many ways a false dichotomy, and that clinicians can work entirely within the scope of ASHA prescriptions while taking selective inspiration from the lively and multifaceted field of psychotherapy. Indeed, many of the creative methods described and illustrated later in this book do just this, drawing on the spirit or techniques of two kindred perspectives in particular—constructivism and narrative therapy—to offer principles and practices that can give helpful and efficient structure to counseling dimensions of our disciplines. We'll now turn to these perspectives and to their practical implications for working with clients in SLP and audiology settings.

References

Beck, A. T. (1976). *Cognitive therapy and the emotional disorders.* New York, NY: International Universities Press.

Freud, S. (1940). *The standard edition of the complete works of Sigmund Freud.* London, UK: Hogarth.

Messer, S. B., & Gurman, A. S. (Eds.). (2011). *Essential psychotherapies.* New York, NY: Guilford.

Neimeyer, R. A., Kazantzis, N., Kassler, D. M., Baker, K. D., & Fletcher, R. (2008). Group cognitive-behavioral therapy for depression outcomes predicted by willingness to engage in homework, compliance with homework, and cognitive restructuring skill acquisition. *Cognitive Behaviour Therapy, 37*, 199–215.

Rogers, C. R. (1961). *On becoming a person.* Boston, MA: Houghton Mifflin.

Sommers-Flanagan, J., & Sommers-Flanagan, R. (2012). *Counseling and psychotherapy theories in context and practice* (2nd ed.). New York, NY: Wiley.

Westen, D. (1998). The scientific legacy of Sigmund Freud: Toward a psychodynamically informed psychological science. *Psychological Bulletin, 124*, 333–371.

Wolpe, J. (1958). *Psychotherapy by reciprocal inhibition.* Stanford, CA: Stanford University Press.

5

CONSTRUCTIVISM

What is *constructivism*, and why do we believe that it offers a help-ful frame for counseling in the field of communication disorders? At its most basic level, such a perspective focuses on the active process of constructing or making meaning of life experiences, both in deeply personal ways and in interaction with others in the social world. Constructivist counseling therefore focuses on *intervening in meaning*, as well as in helping clients perform new and more adaptive behaviors (Kelly, 1955/1991; Neimeyer, 2009). Such an approach is holistic, in the sense that it gives equal weight to people's feelings and thoughts and to their overt behavior.

Personal Construct Theory

The original constructivist perspective in clinical practice was for-mulated by psychologist George Kelly (1955/1991), who objected both to the unconscious determination of people's destinies em-phasized by psychoanalysts of his day, and to the environmental determinism that characterized early behaviorists. Instead, Kelly viewed the human being as a "form of motion," intrinsically active and inquisitive, each formulating his or her own "theory" of life and testing it out in practical contexts. For example, a student who an-ticipates a fulfilling career in audiology might test this "hypothesis" by interning in an audiology practice, and confirming or modifying her ideas about whether this would be an interesting career path as a result. One of the audacious aspects of Kelly's theory was that this view of life as a kind of "personal science" applies equally to the most "disordered" client as to the most effective professional. For example, an older man with moderate hearing loss might anticipate that going to a noisy restaurant with family and friends would prove challenging or embarrassing as he would struggle to participate in conversation, and hence might avoid eating out, even if this also contributed to marital tensions or social isolation. In this case, no less than that of the professional intern, the person's behavior follows logically from what he or she anticipates, and modifying this behavior, therefore, requires reviewing and revising the associated meanings as well. The case described in Chapter 2 involving Flora and her reluctance to share meals with her family provides a further example of this concept.

The Experience Cycle

Kelly (1955) formalized this process of formulating and testing our personal theories in terms of an *experience cycle* having five stages, which subsequent construct theorists (Neimeyer, 1987; Oades & Viney, 2012) have extended as a clinically useful way of understanding clients and their problems (Figure 5-1). First, Kelly assumed that all behavior was anchored in sometimes explicit, but usually implicit *anticipation*. That is, we usually have some idea or expectation of what a given situation will hold, although we might not realize this until our expectations are violated by something that surprises us! Second, we have varying degrees of *investment* in the outcome. Sometimes the events into which we are thrust or in which we choose to engage matter to us only a little, and other times they matter a great deal. Third, we *encounter* the event. Something happens, and we are forced to take it into account, one way or the other. Fourth, we experience *confirmation or disconfirmation* of our anticipations. Things turn out pretty much as we predicted . . . or very differently, and this can be a perturbing or even threatening experience. Finally, we are prompted to undertake a *constructive revision* of our system. This might amount to

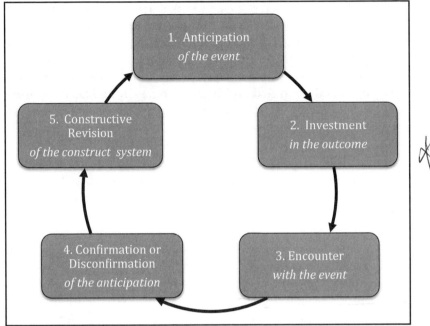

Figure 5–1. The Experience Cycle. Adapted with permission from Neimeyer, R. A. (1987). An orientation to personal construct therapy. In R. A. Neimeyer and G. J. Neimeyer (Eds.), *Personal construct theory casebook* (pp. 3–19). New York, NY: Springer. Reprinted with permission.

believing all the more strongly in our original expectations, or altering them substantially in light of experience. The result shapes our future anticipations in similar situations, and the cycle continues.

How is this cycle useful in the counseling context? The answer is: in several ways. First, it gives the clinician a way to help clients become *connoisseurs of their experience*, to slow down and examine how their anticipations both shape and are shaped by their behavioral encounter with relevant situations. Consider the case of a recently retired gunnery sergeant who was deployed for nearly three years to Iraq. Although not quite 40 years old when he re-entered life as a civilian, he, like many in his position, had experienced a good deal of trauma to his hearing from the seemingly constant exposure to gunfire, mortar barrages, and explosions.

Married, and looking forward to a new career in emergency medicine, he *anticipated* that he would master the classes required in his community college program much as he had the frequent training he had in the army. Moreover, he was highly *invested* in the outcome; with two children to raise and a new career on the horizon, he eagerly enrolled and began classes. But what he *encountered* was initially jarring: he had a hard time hearing the teacher in the large classes, and especially struggled to understand one fairly soft-spoken nurse who was his instructor in wound care. Suddenly, he found himself *disconfirmed* in his expectation that he would breeze through the new curriculum, and began to *revise* his theory of himself along more negative lines, as less capable than he imagined. The resulting anxious anticipation of future classes that still mattered greatly in his program led him to start finding excuses to skip more and more of them, which in turn reinforced his growing sense of inability to handle the program.

Eventually confronted by his wife for his behavior, he was forced to do something about the hearing loss that he had tried to ignore and that ultimately had contributed to his struggles in the classroom. Going over the story of what led him to seek an audiological consultation, the audiologist compassionately asked about what he expected on returning to school, what actually had transpired, and what he made of it. But rather than buying into his self-doubts about his inability as a student, she focused on a dimension of the problem he could do something about—namely, seek a closer seat, assertively ask for the instructor to repeat something when he had trouble hearing it, and, just maybe, consider a hearing aid. In Kelly's terms this intervention was in keeping with his philosophy of *constructive alternativism*: the idea that we are always free to reconstrue, or find new meanings for, that which we cannot deny. Stated differently, it is often useful to consider different interpretations of problem circumstances, as these can often suggest different and more effective conclusions.

But because the clinician's suggested course of action further threatened to disconfirm the veteran's somewhat macho theory of himself as young, strong, and in control, he resisted taking this step until the clinician encouraged him to start noticing how many other young veterans in the clinic also used assistive devices. Eventually striking up conversations with several of them, he underwent another corrective experience cycle, revising his theory that "real men don't need help" in light of these encounters, and ultimately accepting and using a device that greatly improved his comfort and performance in the program, and launched him securely into his new career. This outcome suggests a second use of the experience cycle, to not only help understand problematic experiences, but also to launch new and more effective ones. Chapter 21, *Experimenting with Experience*, further pursues the practical implications of this model in working with communication disorders.

As some of the above examples suggest, to say that clients behave like personal scientists is not to say that they behave like *optimal* scientists, readily seeking out new evidence and modifying their theories accordingly. Indeed, just as professional scientists often build their careers by conducting "safe" studies whose results are likely to confirm, rather than disconfirm their hypotheses, so too clients may behave in such a way that their anticipations, even if uncomfortable in some ways, are validated. For example, a young man who stutters might anticipate social rejection in situations where he is disfluent, and so minimize contact with others where conversation is necessary. Of course, this in turn could lead to his further social disengagement, creating an identity or "way of life" (Fransella, 1972) in which the world of stuttering and avoidance become normal and known, whereas the world of fluency and friendship are perceived as unfamiliar and threatening. Recent research, to be discussed in Chapter 7, lends support to this view, suggesting the relevance of counseling interventions that examine how the client adopts an identity as someone with a problem, and that provide support for constructing and testing new adaptive behaviors.

The Structure of Construct Systems

One of the novel features of personal construct theory has to do with its conceptualization of constructs as *bipolar*—not in the sense of their being manic depressive, but in the sense that they represent a series of opposites, like "popular versus rejected," "young versus old," or "healthy versus ill." That is, *meaning is a matter of contrast*: every affirmation of what someone or something *is*, is also an implicit statement of what someone or something *is not*. Kelly thought of constructs as "reference axes," ways of orienting practically in the world: we need to distinguish between "times to go to bed versus times to get up," tell the difference between "people who like us versus those who don't," and recognize when we are "succeeding versus failing." In a clinical context, this idea helps us tune in to what a client *isn't* saying, as when a student receiving speech therapy in school says she "likes gym class best" (because she doesn't have to speak to other children), or "wants to stay in study hall" (because she doesn't like being embarrassed by being singled out for therapy sessions). Often it is the implied contrast that gives a construct its punch, as, for example, when a client views himself as "a stutterer" (vs. "normal").

A second structural feature of constructs with practical implications is that they form *systems* in which some constructs are more central, or related to the *core*, whereas others are more *peripheral*. Among the most central constructs in our systems, according to Kelly (1955), are our *core role constructs*, those that anchor our most basic sense of identity in the social world. While we might readily enough modify our peripheral constructs, deciding to wear sandals rather than boots on a warmer than expected day, we typically resist change in those core constructs that form the foundations of our sense of self, such as deciding to dress in a sloppy way if we view ourselves as a very neat or controlled person. Accordingly, while small scale and temporary changes in our behavior are relatively easy to accommodate for most people—including those who consult speech-language pathologists and audiologists—more sweeping changes in our basic personality or the image we project to others can be more threatening, more actively resisted, or at least more gradually consolidated.

For example, in the earlier example of the gunnery sergeant, his core construct of himself as "a man" was linked to more peripheral constructs like "not needing help," "not wearing hearing aids," and so on. Understandably, then, he initially resisted shifting to the opposite poles of these constructs by seeking professional assistance and wearing an assistive device, as this seemed to be at odds with his sense of manhood. Only when he began to change his constructs by noticing and speaking with other veterans who had made similar accommodations was he able to consider the behavior change necessary to approach his instructor more assertively and accept the technology that helped him succeed in his program.

Constructs and Emotions

The emphasis on "testing our personal theories" in a constructivist approach to counseling might sound rather intellectual or cognitive, but in fact it can be a profoundly emotional experience. Indeed, Kelly (1955/1991) saw *construing*—the process of applying our meanings to life events and seeking their validation—as an inherently passionate process. From this perspective, human beings are viewed as "wired" to seek to make sense of who they are, what they do, and how others respond to them. When successful, we can experience a range of positive emotions that accompany confirmation of our construing, affirming the contours of our familiar world. Even when our experiences are unpleasant—as when others respond with awkwardness to our customary stuttering, or laugh at our frequently misunderstanding a fragment of conversation we couldn't clearly hear—we at least experience the confirmation of our anticipations, reinforcing our usual ways of dealing with these familiar situations. But when we find ourselves in a situation for which we have few if any constructs to anticipate what will happen next, we may experience severe *anxiety*, in essence being "caught with our constructs down." The voice client referred to in the earlier chapter who was accustomed to using her forceful "cheerleading" voice in most situations could well become anxious when confronted with the need to display unfamiliar behaviors in social situations, such as remaining silent to rest her voice or speaking in a quieter, more breathy fashion. Some clients might even feel a *threat* when coached to present themselves in a way that seems to contradict their usual ways of engaging the world, as when someone who stutters is encouraged to practice public speaking while using new behavioral skills to produce fluent-sounding speech. At the extreme, such clients might even feel *guilt* in Kelly's sense of behaving in a way that clashes with their "true" sense of who they are, believing that they are "deceiving" others by performing in a way that feels artificial (Kelly, 1955/1991). Research that explores these impediments to therapeutic change is further discussed in Chapter 7.

Conclusions

Personal construct theory is a theory of human meaning, one that carries many practical implications for clients when we as professionals are trying to help them face the anxieties that attend all change. As we will see, even the most straightforward of technical interventions can imply substantial adaptive challenges, in the sense discussed in Chapter 3. Constructivist counseling methods are especially valuable in clarifying and addressing such impediments to change, as illustrated in Chapter 7 and the many "toolbox" chapters to follow.

References

Fransella, F. (1972). *Personal change and reconstruction*. London, UK: Academic.

Kelly, G. A. (1955/1991). *The psychology of personal constructs*. New York, NY: Routledge.

Neimeyer, R. A. (1987). An orientation to personal construct therapy. In R. A. Neimeyer & G. J. Neimeyer (Eds.), *Personal construct theory casebook* (pp. 3–19). New York, NY: Springer.

Neimeyer, R. A. (2009). *Constructivist psychotherapy*. London, UK & New York, NY: Routledge.

Oades, L., & Viney, L. (2012). Experience cycle methodology. In P. Caputi, L. L. Viney, & N. Crittenden (Eds.), *Personal construct methodology* (pp. 3–51). New York, NY: Wiley.

6

NARRATIVE THERAPY

As human beings, we live our lives in stories. Over the course of our days, we watch innumerable stories on television, in the movies, and on stage, and read countless more in books, both electronic and paper. More personally, we recount the events of our day to friends and family, just as we reciprocally serve as the audiences for theirs. "Storying" experience, then, seems to come naturally to our species, perhaps to such an extent that we might properly be described as *Homo narrans* rather than *Homo sapiens* (Hermans, 2002).

Among the defining features of narrative activity is that it involves motivated characters, typically animated by some sort of problem whose solution (or its frustration) drives the plot of the story toward some projected end (Neimeyer, 2000). Central to the action is a protagonist who encounters supportive and opposing forces as the narrative unfolds toward a positive outcome (as in a romance or comedy), extended trial (as in an epic or allegory) or a darker conclusion (as in a tragedy or absurdist account). Not surprisingly, we typically cast ourselves, at least implicitly, as the protagonists of most of our story-telling ventures, constructing a tale that usually casts us in a familiar role as hero, problem-solver, comedian, or at least sympathetic victim. And in so doing, across the years we sculpt much of the thematic meaning that our lives will have, as we repeatedly perform our self-narratives and tell them on the stage of the social world (Neimeyer, 2004).

But just as we live our stories, our stories can also come to *live us*. Particularly when we struggle repeatedly with some "problem," especially one that is formally diagnosed as a form of pathology (Foucault, 1970), we can become so identified with the *dominant narrative* of our disorder that we lose any real sense of agency, control, or choice over our lives in the area in which the problem operates (White & Epston, 1990). In a sense we become "colonized" by the story of our brokenness, illness, or deficiency to the extent that at least in traditional (and still quite common) terms we are identified by self and others as "a stutterer," "a laryngectomee," "partially deaf," and other terms that mark us by our diagnosis or difficulty. Narrative therapy (White & Epston, 1990) provides a kind of archeology of such problem-sustaining stories, in the sense of uncovering their origins, and in an act of compassionate defiance, contests their claim as adequate descriptions of the lives they inhabit.

In this brief chapter we sketch the outlines of this approach to counseling, paving the way for the exploration of numerous narrative tools in Part IV of this book, each of which can be creatively adapted to the broad range of challenges confronted by clients who seek consultation for communication disorders.

Deconstructing the Dominant Narrative

In their thoughtful exposition of "story re-vision" in the context of family therapy, Parry and Doan (1994) consider that "the experiences that bring individuals or families to therapy represent, in our view, a "wake-up call"—a message that the stories that have formed them and shaped their emotional reactions have reached their limit" (p. 42). That is, although the story of the client as a person-with-problem may have been sufficient to get them across the threshold of the clinic, it almost by definition fails to help them leave it with a *preferred story* conferring greater adaptation and hope. Instead, that becomes the goal of the treatment team consisting of clinician and client, and the role of narrative therapy is to provide a framework for this effort.

What does this grand idea mean in practice? It means first that the clinician listens for what clients are telling themselves about their disorder or condition, and the extent to which it comes to dominate their view of themselves and their world. Listening between the lines, one can quickly get a sense of how much "space" the problem takes up in the client's life: is it simply an occasional irritant or inconvenience, or is a great deal of the client's time spent wrestling with or avoiding it? It also can be clear by our clients' downward gaze, defensive tone, or reluctance to seek help whether they feel *shamed* by the disorder, as if it diminishes them as a person, or represents a character flaw for which they are ultimately responsible. All of these signs and symptoms—preoccupation with or life-limiting avoidance of the problem, embarrassment or shame, self-disparagement or self-criticism—can all point to the problem as a dominant narrative constraining the client's identity and calling for counseling methods that help *deconstruct* its influence. Several such methods are sketched below and unpacked in considerable detail in later "toolkit" chapters but, basically, "deconstructing" implies that the client and clinician closely examine the dominant narrative of disability or pathology, take it apart to understand how it operates, and actively notice when the client lives and acts beyond the narrow definition of deficiency that it implies. One means by which they can do so is through *externalizing conversations*, a tool to which we now turn.

Externalizing the Problem

Although narrative therapy is inherently flexible, arising as it does from the client's account of his or her experience in interaction with the curious questions of the therapist, in practice certain patterns recur. Often therapy begins with a recitation of the problem story, often related by the client with a sense of reluctance, anxiety, or hopelessness, as if he or she were to blame for the disorder or difficulty. For the narrative therapist, however, the *person* isn't the problem; the *problem* is the problem. The therapist may therefore engage in *relative influence questioning*, first *externalizing* the problem as something separate from the client, and then tracing its influence on him or her over time. Using characteristically colorful questions, the therapist might ask, for example, "When did stuttering first interrupt your conversation with someone? Did stuttering just butt in, or did you see him coming? Did he come and go at first, or did he attach himself to you from that point on? How did you feel about him making his appearance? What plans did he seem to have for your social life?" Interspersing these and similar questions through the interview, the therapist and client would gain a clearer understanding about the problem's influence on the client's past, present, and probable future in a way that clearly distinguishes the disorder from the person who suffers it. In doing so, the person's motivation to resist the dominance of the problem typically builds, and the groundwork is built for deconstructive questions that reverse the focus, and consider the influence of the person on the problem: "Did you ever try to reclaim your own voice in stuttering's interruptive presence? Who or what gives you support in your attempt to do so? Have there ever been times that you've been able to get the best of stuttering? When and how? How might your image of your future be different from the one that stuttering seems to have planned for you?" Here the goal is to "open space for new stories" (Freedman & Combs, 1996), essentially discovering *unique outcomes* or "sparkling moments" when the problem didn't happen, and when the client was able to live out a different identity than the problem-saturated one. By giving these attention, and carefully teasing out how the client resisted the disorder's dominance, the therapeutic team begins a process of "re-visioning" what life might be if lived differently.

Spreading the Good Word

Much of the time problems tend to isolate people, setting them apart from their family or broader community and marking them as "different," "disordered," or "deficient" in some basic skill or ability that is shared by other "normal" people. Accordingly, treatment of the problem tends to be highly private and confidential, much like a Catholic confession of sins to a forgiving priest. Given the shame and guilt that many people with communication disorders experience, the analogy may be uncomfortably apt.

Narrative therapy contests this segregation of the problem person, and instead attempts to build a *community of concern* comprised of supportive others to whom the client can circulate the good news of his or her victories over the problem—a successful class presentation for a student struggling with articulation problems, attendance at a cocktail party or symphony for an adult with hearing loss, a commitment to approach others rather than avoid them. Not uncommonly, the counselor and client might collaborate to share encouraging developments in a letter to the client's supporters, and therapy might conclude with a reception at the clinic that celebrates the client's reclaiming a fuller life that had once been overshadowed by the presence of the problem. All of these steps, and the documentation of successes in overcoming the problem's influence, in effect *thicken the plot* of the new and preferred story of the client as resourceful, competent and resilient, and secure social validation for a less problem-saturated identity. In effect the client leaves therapy with a re-visioned sense of self, and a renewed connection to the social world. Many of the methods described in Part IV of this book can prove useful in the narration and re-narration of client's story, and it is to these that we will turn after a more specific consideration of the implications of constructivism and narrative therapy in the context of the treatment of communication disorders in Chapter 7.

References

Foucault, M. (1970). *The order of things*. New York, NY: Pantheon.

Freedman, J., & Combs, G. (1996). *Narrative therapy*. New York, NY: Norton.

Hermans, H. (2002). The person as a motivated storyteller. In R. A. Neimeyer & G. J. Neimeyer (Eds.), *Advances in personal construct psychology* (Vol. 5, pp. 3–38). Westport, CT: Praeger.

Neimeyer, R. A. (2000). Narrative disruptions in the construction of self. In R. A. Neimeyer & J. D. Raskin (Eds.), *Constructions of disorder: Meaning making frameworks for psychotherapy* (pp. 207–241). Washington, DC: American Psychological Association.

Neimeyer, R. A. (2004). Fostering posttraumatic growth: A narrative contribution. *Psychological Inquiry, 15*, 53–59.

Parry, A., & Doan, R. (1994). *Story re-visions*. New York, NY: Guilford.

White, M., & Epston, D. (1990). *Narrative means to therapeutic ends*. New York, NY: Norton.

7

EVIDENCE FOR A CONSTRUCTIVIST APPROACH TO COUNSELING IN SPEECH-LANGUAGE PATHOLOGY AND AUDIOLOGY

Because clinicians who work with communication disorders are likely to be unfamiliar with a constructivist conceptualization of their field and the evidence suggesting its effectiveness, we review here some of the basic and applied research that reinforces these practices. But before we look at research supporting constructivist and narrative therapy approaches in relation to communication disorders, we want to note the evidence for the efficacy of these approaches to counseling in general, derived from qualitative research such as case studies (e.g., Besa, 1994; Nylund, 2002; Weber, Davis, & McPhie, 2006), ethnographic research (e.g., St. James-O'Connor,

Meakes, Pickering, & Schuman, 1997), and illustrative cases presented as part of a description for treatment of a particular problem (e.g., Madigan & Goldner, 1998; Winslade & Smith, 1997). In addition, conventional quantitative studies using relevant control groups (e.g., Karst & Trexler, 1970; Winter, Gournay, Metcalf, & Rossotti, 2006) have offered encouragement for personal construct counseling and therapy. For example, Holland and Neimeyer (2009) performed a meta-analysis of 22 quantitative investigations and found support for the efficacy of constructivist interventions, particularly in the management of anxiety, including social anxiety, which has particular relevance for applications in speech-language pathology and audiology.

Personal Construct Psychology and Communication Disorders

Although applying a constructivist perspective to problems in speech-language pathology and audiology appears relatively new, there is a significant amount of research from the 1970's and 1980's in which constructivist approaches were used with clients who stutter, and a growing (recent) evidence base for both its basic premises in communication disorders and for its therapeutic efficacy in other areas of application. Fransella (1972) was the first to connect personal construct psychology (PCP) with stuttering. In her book, *Personal Change and Reconstruction*, Fransella proposed that persons who stutter fail to meaningfully integrate experiences of fluent speech, but, instead, develop construct systems based on the experience of stuttering. She hypothesized that, for persons who stutter, the *fluent-speaker role* tends to lack any meaningful, predictive quality, whereas the *stutterer role* tends to be more "meaningful" in that it facilitates accurate prediction of internal and external reactions to, and consequences of, speaking. Fransella concluded that a person continues to stutter "because it is in this way that he can anticipate the greatest number of events; it is by behaving in this way that life is most meaningful to him" (p. 58). She investigated her claim with 16 persons who stutter (PWS), using a method called the repertory grid to explore their construct (or meaning) systems relative to the stutterer role and fluent-speaker role. Her results supported her hypothesis by indicating significantly more elaborated or extensive systems of constructs related to stuttering than fluent speech for all participants. Fransella and Evesham (1985) then provided evidence for the effectiveness of PCP as part of an overall treatment for stuttering by demonstrating that participants who had been engaged in constructivist counseling as part of a behavioral stuttering treatment program had lower relapse rates than those who received behavioral treatment only.

Building on the work of Fransella, Leahy and Collins (1991) described a group therapy program for adults who stuttered that was based on personal construct psychology. She reported that 5 adult male participants demonstrated increased fluency following the group therapy program. Similarly, Stewart (1996) provided two case examples that demonstrated the efficacy of PCP on the long-term outcomes for PWS and Stewart and Birdsall (2001) described a "client's-eye view" of PCP with a PWS, with a description of how therapy encouraged the client to take "the first steps in elaborating a new identity" (p. 224).

In our own research (DiLollo, Manning & Neimeyer, 2003, 2005), we have investigated the theory that persons who stutter fail to construe any production of fluent speech as meaningful, thereby failing to develop elaborate construct systems related to a fluent speaker role. In one investigation (DiLollo et al., 2003), we conducted a systematic content analytic study that examined the cognitive anxiety (Viney & Westbrook, 1976) of 29 persons who stutter and 29 fluent speakers with respect to "fluent" and "stutterer" speaker roles. Cognitive anxiety may be defined as the inability to *meaningfully integrate* an experience, or, in PCP terms, the awareness that one's construct systems are inadequate to allow full and meaningful construing (and, therefore, prediction) of the events with which the person is confronted (Viney & Westbrook). In this study, the persons who stutter and fluent speakers were interviewed and asked identical, open ended questions regarding what life was like as: (a) a person who stutters and (b) a fluent speaker. Responses to these two questions were transcribed and analyzed using a modified version of Viney and Westbrook's (1976)

Cognitive Anxiety Scale. Results indicated that both persons who stutter and fluent speakers demonstrated significantly higher levels of cognitive anxiety related to their "non-dominant" speaker role compared to their "dominant" role. In doing this, both groups dismissed experiences of the non-dominant role as meaningless, easily glossing over or making excuses for any behavior (i.e., fluent or disfluent speech) that did not match their dominant speaker role. In other words, both groups tightened their constructs and constricted their perceptual fields, construing speech experiences other than those of their dominant speaker role as outside the range of convenience of their construct systems, thus extracting little meaning from those experiences. These findings suggest that such "protection" of the dominant speaker role could become a significant barrier to successful long-term treatment of stuttering if treatment focused only on behavior change. Interestingly, subsequent qualitative research on the long-term successful management of stuttering suggests that those who substantially overcome stuttering consciously struggle to reorganize a sense of self in the wake of speech fluency improvement (Plexico, Manning, & DiLollo, 2010).

A second study involved the same 29 PWS who participated in the previously described cognitive anxiety study. For this study (DiLollo et al., 2005), we re-analyzed the transcripts from the PWS by applying a measure of *cognitive complexity* (Bieri, 1955; Crockett, 1965) to examine the relative meaningfulness of the fluent speaker role compared to the "stutterer" role. Cognitive complexity may be defined as the degree of differentiation (i.e., number of different constructs) in an individual's construct system. According to Crockett, the number of constructs participants use to describe a specific domain of interest will be a reflection of the complexity of their construct system with respect to that domain. In this study, the number of constructs used by PWS to describe the domains of their *fluent speaker role* and their *stutterer role* were taken to indicate the cognitive complexity—or meaningfulness—of each of those speaker roles. Participants in this study demonstrated significantly less complex construct systems related to the fluent speaker role compared to the stutterer role. These results provided support for the hypothesis that PWS struggle with developing a meaningful fluent-speaker role, despite frequent experiences with fluent speech production.

Although the studies reported on so far have all focused on stuttering, it is not difficult to generalize these findings to the problems that may be encountered by clients with any communication disorder. A client who is attempting to change some aspect of him or herself, as all clients who seek treatment for a communication disorder are, may struggle with making sense of a non-dominant role and taking on a new, different role as a communicator. In fact, Dalton (1988, 1994) described the use of personal construct psychology as a way for speech-language pathologists to work with clients with *any* communication disorder. She explored the effects that communication disorders can have on persons' sense of self, relationships, and perceptions of the world, and regarded the clinician's ability to better understand the lives of clients as paramount to successful treatment. An example of just such an application of personal construct psychology was reported by Cunningham (1998). She used the principles of personal construct psychology and repertory grids to engage an 89-year-old male with severe aphasia in counseling. Cunningham reported that the counseling and repertory grids provided a structure that helped the client explore how he viewed important parts of his life and resulted in improved quality of life.

Sechtem (2013) also echoed Dalton's (1988, 1994) conclusions in a study involving persons with aphasia and their communication partners. He investigated the influence of three communication partner variables (of which cognitive complexity was one) on conversational effectiveness following training in supported conversation (Kagan, 1999). In this case, cognitive complexity was being used as a measure of the complexity of the communication partners' construct system related to communication, with the assumption that more complex systems would allow for more effective learning of the supported conversation techniques. Pre- and post-training 10-minute conversations were videotaped and analyzed using adapted versions of Kagan's supported conversation scales, which rate the effectiveness of the conversations. Results indicated increased post-training conversational effectiveness for all participants, but no significant correlation between cognitive complexity and the conversational effectiveness of trained communication partners. Sechtem did, however, find a significant correlation between partner cognitive complexity and the conversational effectiveness of the person with aphasia. This finding suggested that communication partners with higher levels of cognitive complexity were able to more effectively interact with the person with aphasia to get them to produce richer, more complex communications, despite there being no significant difference in specific techniques used. What is significant about this finding is that it demonstrates the importance of more subtle facets of communication that relate to aspects of "connectedness" and "meaning" rather than simple behaviors and application of techniques. It also suggests that counseling the communication partner—often a spouse or adult child—to help him or her develop a more empathic understanding of the feelings, frustrations, and functional skills of the aphasic family member (that is, a more complex and nuanced construct system of the patient) could help the communication partner to effectively encourage more complex and satisfying communication.

Additionally, research driven by a constructivist philosophy has emerged from the field of audiology. For example, Kelly, Neimeyer, and Wark (2011) investigated cognitive anxiety in relation to hearing loss. They studied the decision to consult for hearing services on the part of 93 older adults living in the community and found that cognitive anxiety was *highest* among those who were consulting audiologists for the first time, and *lowest* among those who had completed the evaluation and had been fitted with assistive devices, with hearing-impaired adults living without hearing aids being in between these two groups. These findings reflect the role of the construct system in promoting personal change. The participants in this study who demonstrated the highest level of cognitive anxiety—or inability to adequately construe their situation—were driven to seek an audiologic consultation, whereas those for whom the level of cognitive anxiety was not as high appeared willing to continue living without hearing aids. And in keeping with our understanding of cognitive anxiety, those who had already been fitted with aids demonstrated the lowest cognitive anxiety because they were already building more constructs relative to this domain—in essence, drawing fresh "maps" of the terrain of a new life with expanded hearing.

Similarly, Parry (2013) also used the cognitive anxiety measure with 25 hearing-impaired individuals who were consulting an audiologist for the first time. Results indicated a significant relationship between level of hearing loss and cognitive anxiety, suggesting that cognitive anxiety is higher for those with greater difficulty hearing, particularly in relation to hearing speech. Furthermore, cognitive anxiety was also shown to be significantly higher for participants who reported a lower quality of life. These findings support the previous suggestion by Kelly et al. (2011) that higher cognitive anxiety may be associated with the decision to seek help for a communication problem. The convergence of such findings across different research groups and different samples of clients provides further support for the robustness of these results, and encourages closer study of these processes in future research.

Narrative Therapy and Communication Disorders

As consequence of our work with PCP, we recognized the usefulness in incorporating concepts about how people construct identity and make sense of, and give meaning to, experience into treatments for communication disorders. We also, however, recognized that formal training in personal construct therapy was not a realistic goal for most speech-language pathologists or audiologists, and, without such training, clinicians may be reluctant to embrace such an approach. Consequently, we suggested that an approach such as narrative therapy, still grounded in constructivist principles but more "conversational" in implementation, might be a better fit for speech-language pathologists and audiologists to use as a base for their counseling strategies (DiLollo, Neimeyer, & Manning, 2002).

Following the recommendations made in our 2002 article (DiLollo et al., 2002), a number of authors have reported on the use of narrative therapy with persons who stutter. Leahy and Warren (2007) reported on the use of narrative therapy with a man who was searching for a way to better manage his stuttering. Although leading a confident, successful life, the client viewed stuttering as a "burden" that interfered with how he wanted to be as a person in all facets of his life. The client described a history of successfully controlling stuttering following treatment, but also that stuttering always seemed to reassert itself sometime later. Leahy and Warren described the process of externalizing the problem, referring to it as the "stammering entity," and how it was "out to get" him and that it had "power over" him. By considering a series of questions such as, "What would happen if you had equal power?" and "How can you get that feeling of equal power?" possibilities for changes in thinking were created. The client also gave a voice to the stuttering, writing the narrative of its journey with him—an activity similar to the "autobiography of the problem" tool described in Chapter 15. The clinician and client used this autobiography of stuttering to examine the relationship between stuttering and the client and to determine facets of that relationship that needed to change if successful long-term management of stuttering was to be achieved. Through this re-authoring of his relationship with stuttering, the client was able to take control and to begin to envision a personal narrative where the "stuttering entity" played an increasingly smaller role.

Logan (2007) and Leahy, O'Dwyer, and Ryan (2012) also reported on the successful use of narrative therapy with clients. These reports specifically focused on the power of using "outsider witnesses" (such as the client's friends or family members) as a way for clinicians to co-author new and preferred identities with their clients. As described in Chapter 6, personal narratives are formed within social, political, and cultural contexts and, therefore, any emerging alternative narratives need to also include such contexts. The concept of "outsider witnesses" was developed by White (2004) to promote clients' engaging more fully with their preferred identity while also having the story acknowledged and legitimized by an audience. This public telling and the audience's response and re-telling of the alternative story can have a powerful grounding effect for the client.

Logan (2007) reported a case in which outsider witnesses were used to facilitate the development of an alternative, preferred identity for an adult, male PWS who had recently completed an intensive behavioral stuttering treatment program. In this case, the client's story was video recorded and played for other PWS, and their responses were video recorded and shared with the client. When showing the client's story to the other PWS (outsider witnesses), the clinician asked them to consider four kinds of responses described by White (2007) that included: (1) identifying the expression or what captured your imagination, (2) describing images that the client's story evoked, (3) embodying responses or what resonated with your own life, and (4) acknowledging transport or how you were moved as a result of witnessing the story. Finally, the "re-telling of the re-telling" (p. 328) occurs when the client responds (in this case to the therapist) to the witness' responses to his story. For the client in this study, the re-authoring of his story of stuttering as being less influential in his life was substantiated and supported by the outsider witness process.

Similarly, Leahy et al. (2012) reported on a case of a female adult PWS who engaged in a "definitional ceremony" that included family members and provided her with a way of presenting herself in different and preferred ways. White (1995) adopted Myerhoff's (1982) concept of "definitional ceremonies" as a metaphor for the work that he was doing with encouraging clients to "be active participants in their own history" and the role that he saw in treatment for reflecting teamwork. For White, the definitional ceremony had four parts: (1) a conversation between the client and clinician, observed by the outsider witnesses; (2) a conversation among the witnesses (about what they just saw), observed by the client and clinician; (3) a second conversation between client and clinician, reflecting on the first conversation and the conversation of the witnesses, also observed by the witnesses, and, finally, (4) a debriefing conversation involving client, clinician, and witnesses. The definitional ceremony reported by Leahy et al. was video recorded, transcribed, and analyzed using a hermeneutic phenomenological approach. Findings indicated that the process of the definitional ceremony aided in the expansion and grounding of a preferred story for the participant, and highlighted the importance of including significant others in therapy.

McCormack (2011) reported on the incorporation of narrative therapy into a treatment program for adults who stutter. The *Free to Stutter . . . Free to Speak* (FTS . . . FTS) program is a week-long, intensive program that combines traditional speech therapy treatment with narrative therapy and mindfulness, with the additional use of art to aid the PWS in the free expression of his or her personal experience. McCormack gathered qualitative data from participants through a group interview and a focus group discussion that followed the treatment program. Results of the study indicated significant reductions in feelings of shame, helplessness, and fear of social penalty that had characterized the participants prior to the treatment program and a re-authoring process that led participants to an identity that acknowledged the presence of stuttering, but resisted its dominance and control over their life choices. The researchers and clients identified the narrative therapy component as being central to this re-authoring process.

In addition to these studies related to stuttering, a number of other studies have demonstrated the efficacy of a narrative therapy approach with clients with other communication disorders. For example, Wolter, DiLollo, and Apel (2006) describe the use of a narrative therapy approach with Anna, a 22-year-old woman with language-literacy deficits, and how this approach helped the client develop more effective strategies for coping with her problem and to begin the process of re-authoring her personal narrative. For example, Wolter et al. described the use of externalizing language (see Chapters 8 and 11 for more on *externalizing*) with Anna and described how, by seeing the problem (she called it "LD") as external to herself, Anna was able to join with the clinician to resist LD's influence more effectively than she had in the past. Furthermore, through a series of questions designed to explore alternative storylines and futuremore, possibilities (see *Relative Influence Questions* and *Unique Outcome Questions* in Chapter 10), Anna was able to envision a future in which LD did not dominate and control her.

Similarly, Barrow (2008) explored the culturally imposed dominant narratives of "disability" and their impact on how Anne, a woman with aphasia, and her family made sense of the world. These narratives included "limited competence," "passive role," "disability as less than whole," "restitution," and "chaos." For Anne and her family, a dominant narrative of "restitution" guided behaviors and decisions, despite suggestions from health care professionals that pre-stroke levels of speech would not be regained. Barrow described how collaboratively searching for alternative narratives of disability through active listening, identifying "unique outcomes" (see Chapters 8 and 10 for more on unique outcomes or what we have termed *iMoments*), connecting with others, and creative use of pictures and other media, could help to increase the client's quality of life.

In the field of audiology, DiLollo, DiLollo, English, Mendel, and McCarthy (2006) describe a narrative therapy approach, using composite case studies to illustrate the advantages to listening and responding to a client's story when working with clients with acquired hearing loss. Nelson Crowell, Hanenburg, and Gilbertson (2009) and Harvey (2009) also describe the use of narrative therapy with clients with hearing loss, but at different stages of the life span. Crowell et al, describe successfully using narrative therapy with adolescents with hearing loss. They reported that teens with hearing loss can often be "fixated" on a problem-saturated narrative that negatively affects their self-esteem. Through a joint effort on the part of the clinician and the client, narrative therapy can help these adolescents find an alternative, richer, and more empowering narrative.

Harvey (2009), on the other hand, described the case of an elderly male who was struggling with accepting the substantial editing of his personal narrative by his encroaching hearing loss. Harvey engaged the client in an externalizing activity in which he "interviewed" the hearing loss. Over a number of sessions, the clinician and client (and the hearing loss) discussed ways in which the hearing loss had controlled the client's life and ways in which it had failed to do so. As this process unfolded, the client's story began to shift from one of a "loser" to one of "sometimes a fighter" (p.118). Taking this as a clue to a potential alternative story, Harvey suggested a further interview, this time with the client's long-since dead grandfather (see Chapter 22, *Chair Work* for more on this), a military man whom the client greatly admired. The result of this process was that the client, with the support of his wife and grandfather, formulated a "battle plan" that moved the client toward both "technical" and "adaptive" changes needed to successfully deal with his hearing loss.

Finally, there has been recent interest in the application of narrative therapy with older children and adolescents with autism. Cashin (2008) suggests that externalization techniques might be useful in working with adolescents with Asperger's disorder. He reports on the successful use of such an approach with a 13-year-old boy with Asperger's who was having severe difficulties with anger and aggressive behavior at school. Similarly, Cashin, Browne, Bradbury, and Mulder (2013) report on a pilot study to examine the effectiveness of narrative therapy with young people with autism who present with emotional and behavioral problems. Ten young people with autism (aged 10–16 years) received five 1-hour narrative therapy sessions, conducted over 10 weeks. Results indicated a significant reduction in psychological distress (measured through the Kessler-10 scale; Kessler et al., 2002), and emotionality (measured by the *Emotional Symptoms Scale of the Strengths and Difficulties Questionnaire*; Goodman, 1997). Cashin et al. (2013) conclude that narrative therapy has merit as an intervention with young people with autism, and recommended further research on this topic.

Conclusions

The themes that emerge from research on constructivist and narrative therapy approaches to working with clients with communication disorders orient us to important features that should be included as part of the framework for counseling that we will describe in the next chapter. From the constructivist research, it is clear that a central problem for individuals with communication disorders may revolve around a lack of meaningfulness of their nondominant speaker role, and, just as importantly, a protection of their dominant speaker role. This suggests the need for clinicians to help clients reconstrue their roles as communicators in the light of the behavioral changes that occur during traditional speech pathology and audiology treatment sessions and that techniques and processes typically used in personal construct therapy can achieve these goals.

The research on narrative therapy demonstrates that this approach can also be useful in facilitating the types of reconstruing indicated in the constructivist research, but, by the nature of the focus on language and story, may be more conducive to being incorporated into traditional speech pathology and audiology sessions. Furthermore, the narrative therapy feature of *externalizing* appears to be particularly useful for helping clients with communication disorders to find ways of resisting the effects of their problem and begin viewing themselves in ways that promote more preferred identities.

Finally, both constructivist and narrative therapy approaches promote client-centered thinking and focus on fostering a strong client–clinician alliance. This aspect has been identified as a primary factor in the process of change (e.g., Wampold, 2001) and the success of traditional interventions (e.g., Plexico, Manning, & DiLollo, 2010).

In summary, a growing literature appearing in several peer-reviewed publications and across different disorders is beginning to advance the relevance of a narrative constructivist perspective for counseling conducted by SLPs and audiologists. This body of basic and applied research provides encouragement for greater use of constructivist models and narrative methods in the field of communication disorders. In a sense, this book is written to help professionals in our field take a step in both directions, by discussing clear principles and procedures that facilitate further research on the efficacy of this perspective, and its implementation in concrete clinical contexts. It is to this task that we turn in the next chapter.

References

Barrow, R. (2008). Listening to the voice of living life with aphasia: Anne's story. *International Journal of Communication Disorders, 43*, 30–46.

Besa, D. (1994). Evaluating narrative family therapy using single-system research designs. *Research on Social Work Practice, 4*(3), 309–325. doi:10.1177/104973159400400303

Bieri, J. (1955). Cognitive complexity-simplicity and predictive behavior. *The Journal of Abnormal and Social Psychology, 51*(2), 263–268. doi:10.1037/h0043308

Cashin, A. (2008). Narrative therapy: A psychotherapeutic approach in the treatment of adolescents with Asperger's disorder. *Journal of Child and Adolescent Psychiatric Nursing, 21*(1), 48–56. doi:10.1111/j.1744-6171.2008.00128.x

Cashin, A., Browne, G., Bradbury, J., & Mulder, A. (2013). The effectiveness of narrative therapy with young people with autism. *Journal of*

Child and Adolescent Psychiatric Nursing, 26(1), 32–41. doi:10.1111/jcap.12020

Crockett, W. H. (1965). Cognitive complexity and impression formation. In B. A. Maher (Ed.), *Progress in experimental personality research* (Vol. 2, pp. 47–90). New York, NY: Academic Press.

Cunningham, R. (1998). Counseling someone with severe aphasia: An explorative case study. *Disability and Rehabilitation, 20*, 346–354.

Dalton, P. (1988). Personal construct psychology and speech therapy in Britain: A time of transition. In G. Dunnett (Ed.), *Working with people: Clinical uses of personal construct psychology* (pp. 54–67). Florence, KY: Taylor & Francis.

Dalton, P. (1994). *Counselling people with communication problems.* Thousand Oaks, CA: Sage.

DiLollo, A., Manning, W.H., & Neimeyer, R. A. (2003). Cognitive anxiety as a function of speaker role for fluent speakers and person who stutter. *Journal of Fluency Disorders, 28*(3), 167–186. doi:10.1016/S0094-730X(03)00043-3

DiLollo, A., Manning, W. H., & Neimeyer, R. A. (2005). Cognitive complexity as a function of speaker role for adult persons who stutter. *Journal of Constructivist Psychology, 18*(3), 215–236. doi:10.1080/10720530590948773

DiLollo, A., Neimeyer, R. A., & Manning, W. H. (2002). A personal construct psychology view of relapse: Indications for a narrative therapy component to stuttering treatment. *Journal of Fluency Disorders, 27*(1), 19–42. doi:10.1016/S0094-730X(01)00109-7

DiLollo, L. D., DiLollo, A., Mendel, L., English, K., & McCarthy, P. (2006). Facilitating ownership of acquired hearing loss: A narrative therapy approach. *Journal of the Academy of Rehabilitative Audiology, 39*, 49–67.

Evesham, M., & Fransella, F. (1985). Stuttering relapse: The effect of a combined speech and psychological reconstruction programme. *British Journal of Disorders of Communication, 20*(3), 237–248. doi:10.3109/13682828509012265

Fransella, F. (1972). *Personal change and reconstruction: Research on treatment of stuttering.* Oxford, UK: Academic Press.

Goodman, R. (1997). The strengths and difficulties questionnaire: A research note. *Child Psychology & Psychiatry & Allied Disciplines, 38*(5), 581–586. doi:10.1111/j.1469-7610.1997.tb01545.x

Harvey, M. A. (2009). Preparing for battle against the hearing loss: A narrative therapy approach. *Journal of the American Deafness and Rehabilitation Association, 42*, 114–127.

Holland, J. M., & Neimeyer, R. A. (2009). The efficacy of personal construct therapy as a function of the type and severity of the presenting problem. *Journal of Constructivist Psychology, 22*(2), 170–185. doi:10.1080/10720530802675904

Kagan, A. (1999). *Supported conversation for adults with aphasia (SCA): Methods and evaluation* (Doctoral thesis). University of Toronto, Toronto, Canada). Retrieved from http://hdl.handle.net/1807/12973

Karst, T. O., & Trexlar, L. D. (1970). Initial study using fixed-role and rational-emotive therapy in treating public-speaking anxiety. *Journal of Consulting and Clinical Psychoogy, 34*(3), 360–366. doi:10.1037/h0029344

Kelly, R. J., Neimeyer, R. A., & Wark, D. J. (2011). Cognitive anxiety and the decision to seek services for hearing problems. *Journal of Constructivist Psychology, 24*(2), 168–179. doi:10.1080/10720531003799691

Kessler, R. C., Andrews, G. G., Colpe, L. J., Hirip, E. E., Mroczek, D. K., Normand, S. T., . . . Zaslavsky, A.M. (2002). Short screening scales to monitor population prevalences and trends in non-specific psychological distress. *Psychological Medicine, 32*(6), 956–976. doi:10.1017/S0033291702006074

Leahy, M. M., & Collins, G. (1991). Therapy for stuttering: Experimenting with experimenting. *Irish Journal of Psychological Medicine, 8*, 37–39.

Leahy, M. M., O'Dwyer, M., & Ryan, F. (2012). Witnessing stories: Definitional ceremonies in narrative therapy with adults who stutter. *Journal of Fluency Disorders, 37*(4), 234–241. doi:10.1016/j.jfludis.2012.03.001

Leahy, M., & Warren, A. (2007). Making stuttering manageable: The use of narrative therapy. In J. Au-Yeung & M. M. Leahy (Eds.), *Research, treatment and self-help in fluency disorders: New horizons. Proceedings of the 5th World Congress on Fluency Disorders* (pp. 320–324). Dublin, Ireland: International Fluency Association.

Logan, J. (2007). From client to consultant: Developing "outsider–witness practices" with adults who stammer. In J. Au-Yeung, & M. M. Leahy (Eds.), *Research, treatment and self-help in fluency disorders: New horizons. Proceedings of the 5th World Congress on Fluency Disorders* (pp. 325–332). Dublin, Ireland: International Fluency Association.

Madigan, S. P., & Goldner, E. M. (1998). A narrative approach to anorexia: Discourse reflexivity, and questions. In M. F. Hoyt (Ed.), *The handbook of constructive therapies: Innovative approaches from leading practitioners* (pp. 380–400). San Francisco, CA: Jossey-Bass.

McCormack, J. (2011). *The experience of people who stutter in a therapy programme using art* (Master's thesis). Dublin City University, Dublin, Ireland.

Myerhoff, B. (1982). Life history among the elderly: Performance, visibility, and remembering. In J. Ruby (Ed.), *A crack in the mirror: Reflexive perspective in anthropology* (pp. 99–117). Philadelphia, PA: University of Pennsylvania Press.

Nelson Crowell, R. L., Hanenburg, J., & Gilbertson, A. (2009). Counseling adolescents with hearing loss using a narrative therapy approach. *Perspectives on Administration and Supervision, 19*, 72–78.

Nylund, D. (2002). Poetic means to anti-anorexic. *Journal of Systemic Therapies, 21*(14), 18–34. doi:10.1521/jsyt.21.4.18.23323

Parry, D. C. (2013). *Relationship between cognitive anxiety level and client variables at first consultation for adults with hearing impairment* (Master's thesis). University of Canterbury, Christchurch, NZ.

Plexico, L. W., Manning, W. H., & DiLollo, A. (2010). Client perceptions of effective and ineffective therapeutic alliances during treatment for stuttering. *Journal of Fluency Disorders, 35*(4), 333–354. doi:10.1016/j.jfludis.2010.07.001

Sechtem, P. (2013). *Communication partner variables that influence supported conversation outcomes in aphasia* (Doctoral dissertation). Wichita State University, Wichita, Kansas.

St. James-O'Connor, T., Meakes, E., Pickering, R., & Schuman, M. (1997). On the right track: Client experience of narrative therapy. *Contemporary Family Therapy: An International Journal, 19*(4), 479–495. doi:10.1023/A:1026126903912

Stewart, T. (1996). Good maintainers and poor maintainers: A personal construct approach to an old problem. *Journal of Fluency Disorders, 21*(1), 33–48. doi:10.1016/0094-730X(95)00043-7

Stewart, T., & Birdsall, M. (2001). A review of the contribution of personal construct psychology to stammering therapy. *Journal of Constructivist Psychology, 14*(3), 215–226. doi:10.1080/10720530151143557

Viney, L. L., & Westbrook, M. T. (1976). Cognitive anxiety: A method of content analysis for verbal samples. *Journal of Personality Assessment, 40*(2), 140–150. doi:10.1207/s15327752jpa4002_5

Wampold, B. E. (2001). Contextualizing psychotherapy as a healing practice: Culture, history, and methods. *Applied & Preventive Psychology, 10*(2), 69–86.

Weber, M., Davis, K., & McPhie, L. (2006). Narrative therapy, eating disorders and groups: Enhancing outcomes in rural NSW. *Australian Social Work, 59*(4), 391–405. doi:10.1080/03124070600985970

White, M. (2004). Working with people who are suffering the consequences of multiple trauma: A narrative perspective. *International Journal of Narrative Therapy and Community Work, 1*, 45-76.

White, M. (2007). *Maps of narrative practice.* New York, NY: Norton.

Winslade, J., & Smith, L. (1997). Countering alcoholic narratives. In G. Monk, J. Winslade, K. Crocket, D. Epston (Eds.), *Narrative therapy in practice: The archaeology of hope* (pp. 158-192). San Francisco, CA: Jossey-Bass.

Winter, D., Gournay, K., Metcalfe, C., & Rossotti, N. (2006). Expanding agoraphobics' horizons: An investigation of the effectiveness of a personal construct psychotherapy intervention. *Journal of Constructivist Psychology, 19*(1), 1-29. doi:10.1080/10720530500311141

Wolter, J. A., DiLollo, A., & Apel, K. (2006). A narrative therapy approach to counseling: A model for working with adolescents and adults with language-literacy deficits. *Language, Speech, and Hearing Services in Schools, 37*(3), 168-177. doi:10.1044/0161-1461(2006/019)

8

A THEORY-BASED FRAMEWORK FOR COUNSELING

As we established in Chapter 1, speech-language pathologists (SLPs) and audiologists are contractually and ethically bound to engage in counseling with clients in relation to their speech, language, or hearing problems. The problem for most SLPs and audiologists in counseling clients, however, is that they often have no systematic approach and don't know how to facilitate the types of conversations that will help their clients generate solutions to their problems.

In our own work as counselors and in our many years of experience teaching counseling to speech-language pathology and audiology graduate students, we've discovered that engaging in counseling without a guiding conceptual framework can lead to frustration and feelings of inadequacy; once our preferred technique (which is sometimes more like a "shot in the dark" or, even, no technique at all!) doesn't work, we have no larger frame to resort to in order to figure out why, or to decide where to go next.

These experiences have convinced us that clinicians have two basic needs if they are to counsel clients and feel successful; (1) a theory-based framework that can guide the way they conceptualize their clients and clients' problems, and (2) specific ways to engage clients in counseling conversations that co-construct solutions to those problems. With these two needs met, clinicians can counsel *any clients*, in *any context*. In this chapter we take a look at the theory-based framework that you will need to conceptualize and organize your counseling. In Part IV of this book you will find a series of tools that you can use to facilitate conversations and exercises for engaging clients in counseling, ultimately helping them embrace change.

The Common Factors Model and What It Tells Us About Counseling

In the field of psychotherapy, of which counseling is a part, there are hundreds of distinct approaches that have been described in over 10,000 textbooks (Wampold, 2001), and the number keeps growing every year. So the question then becomes, which of these approaches has been shown to be the most efficacious? The answer, interestingly, is all of them! Wampold and his colleagues (Ahn & Wampold, 2001; Wampold, 2001; Wampold et al., 1997) studied a wide array of psychotherapeutic approaches, trying to identify which approaches had been demonstrated to be superior. What they found was that almost all of the approaches studied were highly effective, suggesting that the specific techniques and processes associated with the various treatments had little to do with the benefits received by the clients. In fact, Wampold and his colleagues calculated that specific treatment ingredients accounted for only 1% of the variation in outcomes. Furthermore, they also found that using a treatment manual that guides the clinician through a specific process of therapy not only did *not* increase benefits but, instead, tended to have a detrimental effect on outcomes by interfering with the development of the client–clinician relationship.

So, what are the "ingredients" for an effective approach to counseling? Wampold (2001) identified a number of "common factors" that appeared to contribute to effective outcomes, regardless of the specific approach that was adopted. These included: (1) the quality of the clinician, (2) clinician allegiance to, or belief in, the treatment protocol, and (3) the nature of the working alliance between the client and clinician. Recent comprehensive reviews of hundreds of controlled studies of treatments for both adults and children strongly reinforce these conclusions (Norcross, 2011). What this research means for clinicians is that provided you adopt an approach that has a sound theoretical base, your job is to: (1) learn as much as you can about the approach you have chosen and how it makes you a better clinician, (2) believe in what you are doing (i.e., the approach you have selected) and stick with the plan, and (3) always pay attention to, and spend time investing in, the therapeutic relationship with your client.

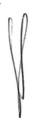

A Constructivist Framework for Counseling Individuals with Communication Disorders and Their Families

In Chapter 2 we discussed the various levels of counseling that might apply in the practice of speech-language pathology and audiology and then in Chapter 3 we discussed the concept of counseling, and therapy in general, as an act of adaptive leadership rather than an act of service. These discussions help us to understand what effective counseling might mean in the context of our two professions: *an overarching framework from which we understand clients and their problems in an adaptive, holistic way and that guides us in facilitating clients' journeys towards effective solutions.*

As we saw in Chapter 4, there are many psychotherapeutic approaches that we might choose to provide such a framework. As you might have guessed from Chapters 5, 6, and 7, we have selected the *constructivist* approach to counseling, of which we consider narrative therapy to be a part, as the theoretical framework for this book. We believe that this constructivist approach: (1) best fits with the concepts of adaptive leadership discussed in Chapter 3, and (2) can be easily integrated into the types of interactions that speech-language pathologists and audiologists already engage in with clients. In the remainder of this chapter, we discuss details of the approach, how it emphasizes the client-clinician relationship, and how to consider it as a *conceptual framework* rather than as a series of prescribed steps.

The idea that this is a *framework* for counseling and not a specific step-by-step process of counseling may make some clinicians nervous. After all, it seems that it would be much easier if we were just told exactly what to do and when and how to do it; then we could be really good counselors! Unfortunately, when dealing with something as complex as the role of communication in the human condition, it is simply not possible to offer a prescribed set of rules or guidelines that will apply to every person in every situation. Try as we might to fit them into our categories, people keep surprising us! If we learn how to conceptualize and understand the human condition, however, then we are much more likely to be able to apply what we know in a creative way with *any client* and in *any situation*. Like improvisational jazz musicians or competitive athletes in a team sport, we then are better poised to take opportunities presented by unpredictable circumstances and carry them forward in progressive directions.

The constructivist framework that we discuss here has five basic principles that will help you to understand your clients and their behaviors (Figure 8–1). These are: (1) the client as expert, (2) personal narratives, (3) alternative ways of construing, (4) innovative moments (or "iMoments"), and (5) co-construction. It is important to remember that these are not "steps" and there is no sequence implied by the numbers. As represented in Figure 8–1, however, the "client as expert" may be viewed as an encompassing "therapeutic stance" (more on that below), with the "personal narrative" as a central concept of the framework. From there, "alternative ways of construing," "iMoments," and "co-construction" feed into personal narrative as ways of helping clients identify and achieve alternative constructions of their personal story.

By understanding these five principles and how they relate to human behavior and motivation, all clinicians should be able to effectively engage their clients in counseling. So, let's now take a look at each of these principles in more detail. Clinicians might like to pay special attention to the "Clinician's Toolkit" boxes that accompany these discussions. These toolkits provide additional information that can help you put the principles into practice.

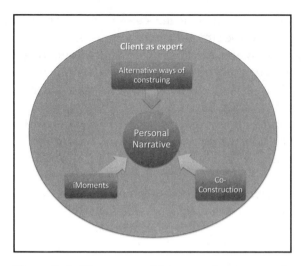

Figure 8–1. The constructivist counseling framework.

Therapeutic Stance: The Client as Expert

Neimeyer (2004) noted that constructivism is "not so much a system of psychotherapy as it is an epistemology, that is, a theory of knowledge." Constructivists believe that knowledge is constructed through interpretation and a search for meaning, that we essentially live in an "interpreted space" between the self and the real world. One implication of this constructivist view is that all knowledge is relative and provisional, even that of professionals and scientists. This further implies that the knowledge that clients possess about their problems may be no less valid and important than the "scientific" knowledge possessed by clinicians. *Consequently, when working within a constructivist framework, clinicians need to "give up" their expert status and role of "problem fixer" and recognize that clients have unique knowledge of the problem and their own personal resources.* As such, clients should be *active* participants in the therapeutic process, not *passive* recipients of the clinician's "expertise." The role of the clinician might be described as that of an interested conversational partner: listening intently, asking curious questions, and taking the client's perspective seriously. One way that clinicians can tell if they are giving up their "expert" status in therapy is to note who is doing most of the talking; in constructivist counseling, at least, it should be the client!

To illustrate this concept, consider the following story from a former client, a young man in his 20's who came to the clinic looking for help with his stuttering: *This young man was very good at avoiding overt stuttering by avoiding feared words and simply not talking much. During his high school years he became extremely distraught about his stuttering, describing himself as feeling "sub-human" and even entertaining thoughts of suicide. He sought help from his school speech-language pathologist, who did her standard testing that revolved around counting his disfluencies and secondary behaviors. At the conclusion of her evaluation, the speech-language pathologist told this young man that*

Clinician's Toolkit #1: The Credulous Approach

As a part of giving up the "expert" role, clinicians need to take up a *credulous approach* as they listen to the problem story told by the client. Raskin and Morano (2004) describe the credulous approach as a stance of openness and acceptance adopted by a clinician in order to understand how the client is presently experiencing the world. The information the client shares in the therapy room is accepted at face value and presumed to be experientially true for that client, even if it does not fit with how others (including the clinician) might construe things.

The credulous approach conveys a great deal of respect for the client's reality, and shows the client that her or his views are valid and valued. *It does not, however, mean that the clinician blindly accepts everything the client says without question.* What is important is that the client feels that his or her problem story has been heard and taken seriously, thereby opening space for therapeutic conversations that focus on alternative ways of construing it.

---

he was not "severe" enough to be in her caseload, so she couldn't help him; he reported that she never even asked him how his stuttering impacted him personally or emotionally as she seemed to think that it was so mild that it should not have been a problem. This is an example of the speech-language pathologist holding onto her "expert" role and not even considering that the client might have a different perspective.

Personal Narratives

We all tell stories about ourselves and our experiences. All you need to do is go to your local Starbucks and you can hear this played out over and over; a huge amount of our communication takes the form of sharing narratives about ourselves with receptive others. What eludes most observers is that there is a two-way influence going on; our stories reflect our self-image but our self-image is also a function of the stories we tell and, as you might recall from Chapter 6, of the stories that others tell about us. Morgan (2000, p. 4) succinctly described this concept, stating that, "As humans, we are interpreting beings. We all have daily experiences of events that we seek to make meaningful. The stories we have about our lives are created through linking certain events together in a particular sequence across a time period, and finding a way of explaining or making sense of them. This meaning forms the plot of the story. We give meanings to our experiences constantly as we live our lives. A narrative is like a thread that weaves the events together, forming a story."

One important aspect of these self-narratives, however, is that only a fraction of our lived experience can be storied and expressed at any one time, resulting in a great deal of life falling outside the dominant stories that form the basis of our self-understanding (White & Epston, 1990). This has important implications for counseling, as it is often in those "glossed over" or ignored experiences that solutions to people's problems reside. As White and Epston (1990) stated, "those aspects of lived experience that fall outside of the dominant story provide a rich and fertile source for the generation, or re-generation, of alternative stories" (p. 15).

Clinician's Toolkit #2: Thin and Thick Descriptions

Allowing the client to take the role of expert and lead therapy is often a problem for SLPs and audiologists, in part because of the tension between using techniques and being person-centered. What aspects of the client's problem require direct "technical" intervention with specific speech, language, or hearing techniques and what aspects require a more person-centered, counseling approach? This is the clinician's dilemma; our role is not entirely that of *counselor* nor is it sufficient for us to merely provide *technical intervention*. Working within a constructivist framework, clinicians pay particular attention to gathering rich, thick descriptions of the client's situation that should help the clinician distinguish these different aspects of the client's problem. (See Chapter 3 for more about technical and adaptive aspects of client's problems.)

Typically, as SLPs and audiologists we are very good at finding out all the relevant details of the speech, language, swallowing, or hearing problem that our clients present. We ask specific questions, often from a list of "standard" case history questions, we use standardized tests, we take speech samples, and we do instrumental testing. All of these activities are important, but all focus solely on the *problem* and not the *person*. One of the basic tenets of this constructivist framework is that the clinician must engage the client in conversations, with the aim of going beyond the "thin description" or, what White (1989) called the "problem-saturated" story, and find a more "thick" description of the person.

"Thin" descriptions derive from a person's unexamined socially and culturally influenced beliefs. These are the descriptions that we get from clients when we ask about the problem. It is the description that extends from the person's dominant self-narrative and is usually limiting and often imposed on us by role stereotypes or what others tell us about who we are.

"Thick" descriptions, on the other hand, more closely correspond to the actuality and complexity of life experienced by the person, and open space for a re-examination of some of the taken-for-granted or "glossed over" moments that may be highly meaningful. Consequently, "thick" descriptions need to be encouraged by clinicians taking a genuine interest in their clients' stories (i.e., not just the problems' story) and, as described earlier, taking the stance that the client is the "expert."

The primary way that clinicians encourage thick descriptions is to ask clarifying and extending questions. DiLollo, Neimeyer, and Manning (2002) used the term "curious questioning" to describe this interaction, with the clinician taking the role of an *interested conversational partner.*

Alternative Ways of Construing

A further implication of the constructivist view of the personal construction of meaning is that alternative constructions of situations are always possible. In more familiar terms, there are always different ways of looking at things. Of course, some interpretations (or ways of construing) may lead to more preferred ways of living than others. For example, if a communication problem is producing emotional and/or social consequences, it is likely that alternative ways of construing that problem or the client's possible identity may prove helpful for clients and their families.

This is not to say that reaching for these new or alternative constructions is easy, however. Evidence of this comes from our research on cognitive anxiety described in Chapter 7. Significantly, we found that all of our participants, both PWS and fluent speakers, had much more "cognitive anxiety" in trying to imagine themselves in their nondominant speaker role than in viewing themselves in their current speaker role (DiLollo, Manning, & Neimeyer, 2003). The significance of this finding is that this lack of ability to construe one's self effectively in an unfamiliar communicative role was not specific to PWS but something that was experienced by essentially "normal" speakers as well, suggesting that this is a reaction that may be an issue for any client, experiencing any type of communication disorder, and receiving any type of technical or behavioral treatment for that disorder. It may seem paradoxical that someone

---

Clinician's Toolkit #3: Externalizing

One way to help clients construe their problem in a different way is by using "externalizing" language. White and Epston (1990) describe externalizing as an approach that "encourages persons to objectify and, at times, to personify the problems that they experience as oppressive. In this process, the problem becomes a separate entity and thus external to the person or relationship that was ascribed as the problem" (p. 38). The effect is to shift the focus of conversation to *the relationship between the person and the problem* rather than on a "problem–person," encouraging greater focus, feelings of control, and options for "dialogue, rather than monologue, about the problem" (p. 40). This enables the clinician and the client to work together to resist the effects of the problem as opposed to the expectation that the clinician will "fix" some broken aspect of the client.

Typically, a single word or short phrase might be used to "name" the problem as way of creating opportunities for the client and clinician to engage in "externalizing conversations." The clinician should always ensure that the name has specific, consistent meaning for the client.

For example, in working with JR, a person who stutters, we decided to use the term "Stuttering" to name his problem. We then tried to incorporate externalizing language in all of our subsequent conversations, talking about how "Stuttering" had "outsmarted" him when he had carefully prepared a presentation for school, practiced it, and was confident of success, only to have a severe block on his name, which he could usually say quite smoothly.

with a communication problem might in some sense resist change, but this often happens when the new world into which therapy would usher them feels unknown and anxiety-producing.

How can clinicians assist clients with the anxiety and perhaps shame of presenting with a problem, as they begin to try to imagine a different life once it is better controlled? One answer is through the use of *externalizing* language (see Chapter 6), which helps clients distinguish the self from the symptom, in a way that lets them view their relation to the problem differently. Clinician's Toolkit #3 offers more details about this useful practice.

Innovative Moments

White and Epston (1990) referred to these aspects of lived experience that fall outside of the dominant story as "unique outcomes." Clinically, these potential alternative storylines may be found in the conversations between the client and clinician that lead to the "thick" descriptions described in the Clinician's Toolkit #2. They show themselves as occasions when the client describes fleetingly overcoming the influence of the problem, dealing with the problem in some creative way, tapping into mostly forgotten personal resources, or even simply forgetting, for a brief moment, that the problem exists.

The challenge for the clinician is to locate these unique outcomes in the "thick" descriptions that emerge from the conversations with the client. Payne (2006) suggests listening for "clues" that the client provides, usually in a passing allusion to some taken-for-granted reference of resistance to the dominant story. An example of a "clue" might be when a client, describing himself as "weak" and "helpless," briefly mentions how he is only able to make it through the day by "cheating" and "bluffing" his way through meetings and lunches so that no one at his office realizes that he has a hearing problem. This might lead to an alternative storyline that focuses on creativity, adaptability, and resourcefulness rather than his current dominant story of helplessness and inadequacy.

Where in the client's story would the clinician look to find evidence of such hopeful steps toward change? One practical guide is provided by Gonçalves and his colleagues (2010), who define unique outcomes in terms of *innovative moments* in therapy (or *iMoments* as we shall call them), a term that may be more apt, as such moments are actually *frequent*, rather than "unique," and reflect the *process* of change more than "outcomes" in the usual sense. In their research, this group has reliably identified five different kinds of iMoments, focused on *protest, reflection, action, reconceptualization,* and *performing change*, which are described more fully in Chapter 10. Higher levels of these iMoments point to good outcomes in therapy of all kinds, including constructivist therapy, which features especially high levels of reflection, leading

---

Clinician's Toolkit #4: Identifying iMoments

Epston and White (1999) suggest a number of questions that might help clients to consider some of the occurrences of resistance or overcoming the effects of the dominant narrative that are taken for granted. Some adapted examples are given here. For more detail on this type of questioning, see Chapter 10.

- Have there been times when you have been able to overcome (*the problem's*) hold over you? How did you feel when this happened?
- How might you stand up to (*the problem*) in the future and refuse its requirements of you?
- What will the future be like without (*the problem's*) influence dominating your life? How is this future different from the one that (*the problem*) would have planned for you?
- Of the people who knew you growing up, who would have been most likely to predict that you would break free from (*the problem's*) influence?
- What qualities would this person have seen in you that would have led him or her to believe that you would have been able to achieve what you have?

to strong reconceptualization and the performance of change over a few sessions (Alves, Mendes, Gonçalves, & Neimeyer, 2012). Being alert to the emergence of different iMoments in counseling tells the clinician that change is occurring, and is available to build on through further interventions like those we will present in future chapters.

Once such iMoments are identified, the client is invited to expand on the circumstances and nature of each, providing as much detail as possible. The clinician again uses "curious questioning" to focus attention on ways in which these events do not fit with the problem-saturated story as previously told. Questioning may include aspects of the person's feelings, thoughts, and actions, and may also invite speculation on how other people who have witnessed these innovative moments might have understood them. In this way, a richer story of the person's life may begin to emerge.

As an example of using iMoments, consider again the story of Mark, presented in Chapter 2. In Mark's story, he talked about being disappointed and surprised about being unable to control his stuttering in a specific situation. As his clinician, I was able to recognize this as a *clue to a potential iMoment* and so asked a series of curious questions about his experience—questions that focused not on his execution of his fluency shaping and modification skills, but on his feelings at the time and the curious aspect of his being surprised by not being able to control stuttering. This iMoment became a significant aspect of Mark's thinking as he moved forward on his therapeutic journey. (See Chapter 9 for more of this conversation with Mark.)

Co-Construction

Recall that we described "thin" descriptions as often imposed on us by role stereotypes or what others tell us about who we are. These are outside influences that play a part in the construction of personal narratives: influences from family, friends, teachers, coworkers, media, gender, racial, and other stereotypes, all of which may contribute to the stories that we author or, more correctly, co-author, about who we are (Winslade & Monk, 1999).

This concept that our stories are essentially "co-authored" by outside influences has certain implications for conducting therapy within a constructivist framework. Firstly, clinicians need to be aware of the stereotypical social, cultural, and political influences that might be contributing to the client's story and actively work to "push back" against such "default" interpretations. Secondly, clinicians must understand their own role in co-authoring the client's story. Working within a constructivist framework, clinicians accept that they *will* play a role in co-authoring the client's story through their interpretation of the client's situation, the questions that they ask, and the re-tellings of the emerging alternative story that they provide. This underscores the importance of clinicians being *client-centered* and their need to guard against imposing their own values and beliefs on the direction that the client's story takes.

Finally, the social construction of self-narratives means that as the client's alternative story begins to emerge, it is important that it be told to others, and told by others, both inside and outside the therapy room. This may involve inviting significant others from the client's life to come to therapy and witness the client's re-telling of the alternative story, or finding "outsiders" to hear and re-tell the story. (See Chapter 10 for more details about using outsider witnesses.) The studies by Logan (2007) and Leahy, O'Dwyer, and Ryan (2012) described in Chapter 7 highlight the power and effectiveness of "outsider witnesses" in facilitating the re-authoring of preferred selves for individuals with communication disorders.

Summary

The constructivist framework described in this chapter requires the clinician to keep in mind five basic principles:

1. The client is the expert and, therefore, should be doing most of the talking, with the clinician acting as a curious conversational partner, eliciting "thick" descriptions from the client that explore the problem in the broader context of the client's life.

2. Think in terms of personal narratives or stories: What story is the client telling and how has the problem influenced the telling of this story?

3. There are always alternative ways of construing the problem, the influences of the problem, and the way that the client is dealing with the problem. One effective way of assisting the client to begin thinking of the problem in a different way is to engage in externalizing conversations.

4. What iMoments can you identify in the client's story? Remember, these are aspects of the client's story that reflect some form of alternative perspective or resistance to the influence of the problem. They are usually just referred to in passing, as they are not yet recognized by the client as *meaningful*. Use specific questions to help the client move forward in this process if needed.

5. The reconstruction of the client's story will involve input from the client, the clinician, and others. It is important for the emerging alternative story to be told and re-told by multiple sources.

The basic processes described in this framework may be incorporated into regular therapy sessions but will require a change in focus from *techniques* to the whole person and his or her lived experience (i.e., adaptive issues). The model presented in Figure 8–2 represents a general conceptual map of therapy that can be applied to any client with any speech, language, hearing, or swallowing disorder. Reading the map from left to right, we can see that a *client* comes to therapy with a speech, language, hearing, or swallowing *problem* and that the problem has two distinct aspects, *technical* and *adaptive*. The technical aspects are the specifics of the speech, language, hearing, or swallowing disorder. The adaptive aspects relate to the impact of those symptoms on the client's quality of life, self-image, and engagement.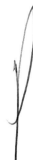

Following the *technical* branch, we see that to address these issues, the clinician takes a *client-centered stance*, with the *clinician as the expert*. From this stance, the clinician applies relevant evidence-based treatment techniques to remediate specific

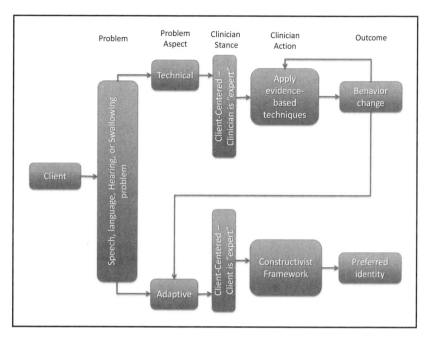

Figure 8–2. A conceptual map of therapy that includes both technical and adaptive branches.

symptoms of the disorder and/or develop effective management strategies. This may be an iterative process that cycles through various techniques to promote behavior change at different levels of complexity. Significantly, however, there is feedback from this technical branch back to the adaptive branch, as the resultant behavior changes carry varying levels of adaptive consequences.

Now following the *adaptive* branch, we see that, as stated above, there is input from *both* the problem and the behavioral changes facilitated by the technical solutions to the problem. To address these issues, the clinician takes a *client-centered stance*, with the *client as the expert*. From this stance, the clinician conceptualizes and engages the client by thinking in terms of the *constructivist counseling framework.* By applying relevant aspects of the framework and associated tools (see Part IV) to the adaptive aspects of the client's problem and the generated behavior changes, the client may emerge with both changes to his or her speech, language, hearing, or swallowing behaviors and a reconstructed, preferred identity that allows for optimal functioning and engagement and improved quality of life.

In the chapters that follow (Chapters 9–12), we look more closely at some of the aspects of the framework and some of the fundamental skills that clinicians will need to develop to improve their counseling with clients and families. We encourage readers to continuously refer back to this basic framework as they read these chapters, with the goal of developing a deeper understanding of the framework how it might and be used to foster adaptive change. We turn first to the most fundamental skills that clinicians need to be successful, not only as counselors, but as clinicians in general: listening and asking questions.

References

Ahn, H., & Wampold, B. E. (2001). Where oh where are the specific ingredients? A meta-analysis of component studies in counseling and psychotherapy. *Journal of Counseling Psychology, 48,* 251–257.

Alves, D., Mendes, I., Gonçalves, M. & Neimeyer, R. A. (2012). Innovative moments in grief therapy: Reconstructing meaning following perinatal death. *Death Studies, 36,* 795–818.

DiLollo, A., Manning, W. H., & Neimeyer, R. A. (2003). Cognitive anxiety as a function of speaker role for fluent speakers and persons who stutter. *Journal of Fluency Disorders, 28,* 167–186.

DiLollo, A., Neimeyer, R. A., & Manning, W. H. (2002). A personal construct psychology view of relapse: Indications for a narrative therapy component to stuttering treatment. *Journal of Fluency Disorders, 27,* 19–42.

Epston, D., & White, M. (1999). Termination as a right of passage: Questioning strategies for a therapy of inclusion. In R. A. Neimeyer, & R. J. Mahoney (Eds.), *Constructivism in psychotherapy*. Washington, DC: American Psychological Association.

Gonçalves, M. M., Santos, A., Matos, M., Salgado, J., Mendes, J., Ribeiro, A., . . . Gonçalves, J. (2010). Innovations in psychotherapy: Tracking the narrative construction of change. In J. D. Raskin, S. K. Bridges, & R. A. Neimeyer (Eds.), *Studies in meaning 4: Constructivist perspectives on theory, practice, and social justice.* New York, NY: Pace University Press.

Leahy, M. M., O'Dwyer, M., & Ryan, F. (2012). Witnessing stories: Definitional ceremonies in narrative therapy with adults who stutter. *Journal of Fluency Disorders, 37*(4), 234-241. doi:10.1016/j.jfludis. 2012.03.001

Logan, J. (2007). From client to consultant: Developing "outsider–witness" practices with adults who stammer. In J. Au-Yeung, & M. M. Leahy (Eds.), *Research, treatment and self-help in fluency disorders: New horizons. Proceedings of the 5th World Congress on Fluency Disorders* (pp. 325-332). Dublin, Ireland: International Fluency Association.

Morgan, A. (2000). *What is narrative therapy? An easy to read introduction.* Adelaide, Australia: Dulwich Center.

Neimeyer, R. A. (2004). Constructivist therapy. In G. R. VandenBos, J. F. McNeil, & S. Reynolds (Executive Producers), *American psychological association series: Systems of psychotherapy.* University Park, IL: Governors State University Communications Services.

Norcross, J. C. (2011). *Psychotherapy relationships that work.* (2nd ed.). New York, NY: Oxford University Press.

Payne, M. (2006). *Narrative therapy: An introduction for counselors* (2nd ed.). Thousand Oaks, CA: Sage Publications.

Raskin, J. D., & Morano, L. A. (2004). Credulous approach. *Internet Encyclopedia of Personal Construct Psychology.* Retrieved September 30, 2011, from http://www.pcp-net.org/encyclopaedia/cred-appr.html

Wampold, B. E. (2001). *The great psychotherapy debate: Models, methods, and findings.* Mahwah, NJ: Lawrence Erlbaum Associates.

Wampold, B. E., Mondin, G. W., Moody, M., Stich, F., Benson, K., & Ahn, H. (1997). A meta-analysis of outcome studies comparing bona fide psychotherapies: Empirically, "All must have prizes." *Psychological Bulletin, 122,* 203-215.

White, M. (1989). *Selected papers.* Adelaide, Australia: Dulwich Center.

White, M., & Epston, D. (1990). *Narrative means to therapeutic ends.* New York, NY: W.W. Norton and Company.

Winslade, J., & Monk, G. (1999). *Narrative counseling in schools: Powerful and brief.* Thousand Oaks, CA: Corwin Press.

Part III

THE PROCESS OF COUNSELING

Over the next five chapters, we revisit aspects of the constructivist framework described in Chapter 8 and take a look at some of the foundational skills that might facilitate clinicians' application of the framework with clients.

9

LISTENING FOR THICK DESCRIPTIONS

No siren did ever so charm the ear of the listener as the
listening ear has charmed the soul of the siren.
Sir Henry Taylor

In the many years that we have been teaching graduate students about counseling, we have observed that one of the primary concerns that students initially bring to class is, "What do I say?" This question identifies one of the fundamental problems that beginning counselors struggle with—thinking that it is about *what they do* and *what they say* that is the essence of counseling—when, in fact, it is just the opposite! As implied by the above quote from Sir Henry Taylor, a 19th century English dramatist and poet, people will talk if we are willing to listen. In this chapter, we explore different types of listening and talk about developing appropriate listening skills. Of course, as counselors, we do engage verbally with our clients, so we also take a look at ways of responding to clients that are client-centered and invite thick, rather than problem-saturated, descriptions of their story.

Listening

Recall that in Chapter 4 we discussed the work of Carl Rogers and the concepts of humanistic psychology that focus on empathy, genuineness, and unconditional positive regard. The therapeutic stance that we described as part of our counseling framework in Chapter 8—the client as expert—fits within this humanistic, client-centered approach to counseling. At the center of such an approach to counseling is the skill of listening. Rogers (1961) believed that simply listening to a client, especially his or her emotions, could lead to positive changes for the client. Similarly, Luterman (2001) stated, "by listening and valuing the client, the professional bolsters the client's confidence so that good decisions are ultimately made" (p. 5). Of course, this concept of "listening," although sounding like something that should be relatively easy—after all, we do this every day—is actually a skill that needs to be shaped and worked on if we are going to use it effectively to encourage our clients to provide thick descriptions.

Inadequate Listening

Let's start out by looking at some of the ways in which we "listen" that are less than adequate. Listening is often confused with hearing, which is simply the act of perceiving sound by the ear and requires little to no effort to accomplish. Listening, on the other hand, requires concentration and focus—something that is not always brought to the table during interactions with others. Egan (2002) described four types of "inadequate listening" that clinicians should pay attention to:

1. *Nonlistening*: This happens when we "tune out"; when we are going through the motions of listening but not really engaging with the other person. We can probably all think of times when we have engaged in nonlistening—aware that someone is talking to us and hearing the sounds that they make but not concentrating enough to actually know what was said or be able to respond appropriately.

2. *Partial listening*: This is listening that "skims the surface," when the listener is only partially engaged and concentrating on what the speaker is saying. It can happen to the clinician if something that the client says triggers a thought or memory about something unrelated to the client's story or if the clinician is engaged in an internal focus on his or her own feelings rather than being present for the client. Thoughts such as, "I wonder what's for dinner tonight?" "Where should we go after work today?" "These shoes really hurt my feet." "I'm really hungry. I need to get some food" or even "This would make a great case study. If things go well, maybe I can write it up and get it published," are examples of distractions that can come up if you are not fully engaged as you "listen" to a client's story.

3. *Tape-recorder listening*: Hearing the words that a client uses to tell her or his story is not the same as listening. Some clinicians reflect back to the client only the words that the client used in talking about an event. Even if you use the exact same words, this is not what the client needs or wants and will not convey to the client that he or she has been listened to. Tape-recorder listening misses out on the deeper meaning and emotion of the message and fails to connect with the client. It reflects a lack of commitment on the part of the clinician to be emotionally and psychologically present for the client.

4. *Rehearsing*: This is a very common problem for clinicians, particularly early in their clinical training or practice. Again, it reflects an internal focus rather than being fully psychologically present for the client. Rehearsing occurs when, during the client's telling of his or her story, the clinician stops listening and starts thinking about, and even rehearsing, how they are going to respond to the client and what questions they will ask. Often, this represents as much a lack of confidence on the part of the clinician as it does a lack of knowledge of how to respond. It also can represent a lack of understanding on the clinician's part of her or his role in the therapeutic process—by holding on to the "expert" role, the clinician assumes the responsibility for having answers and solutions to the client's problems. In contrast, a clinician who has given up that role and made the

client the "expert" has only to engage the client in a way that encourages thick descriptions of the client's problems.

Reflective Listening

The goal for the clinician with regard to listening is what Rogers (1961) termed "reflective listening" but which has also been referred to as "empathic listening" (Egan, 2002), "active listening" (Gordon, 1970), and "empathetic listening" (Luterman, 2001). Regardless of the term used, this form of listening goes beyond merely hearing words and is central to almost any form of humanistic counseling. Rautalinko and Lisper (2004) state that "the purpose of reflective listening is to encourage someone to talk by verifying her or his message in a nonjudgmental fashion" (p. 282). So, by listening in this way, clinicians can encourage the thick descriptions discussed in Chapter 8.

Gordon (1970) defined reflective listening as when someone tries *"to understand what it is the sender is feeling or what his message means. Then he puts his understanding into his own words and feeds it back for the sender's verification"* (p. 50). What Gordon's definition perhaps fails to capture is the intention that, by engaging in this type of listening, there is a change in the therapeutic relationship for *both* the client and the clinician in a positive direction. This change extends from the deep, personal connection that is made, as can be gathered from Rogers' (1980) description of the process of reflective listening: *"It means entering the private perceptual world of the other and becoming thoroughly at home in it. It involves being sensitive, moment by moment, to the changing felt meanings which flow in this other person, to the fear or rage or tenderness or confusion or whatever that he or she is experiencing. It means temporarily living in the other's life, moving about in it delicately without making judgments"* (p. 142).

Luterman (2001), however, warns that if reflective listening is practiced without empathy, a common occurrence for novice clinicians who tend to be more *technique oriented*, then it will fail miserably. Indeed, student clinicians in my counseling class often struggle with this aspect of reflective listening as we initially practice it within the classroom. They use the correct words and even recognize and reflect back feelings embedded within the story told by their partner. For many, however, it is an academic exercise to learn a "technique" and, therefore, they lack to commitment to be psychologically and emotionally present for their partner. Consequently, when debriefing about the activity, some of those who were listened to comment on how "fake" or "condescending" the listener seemed. Many of these students also struggle with wanting to add to or change the message they reflect back, inserting their own opinion, advice, logic, or evaluation of what was said.

Ways of Responding That Invite More Depth from the Client

Rautalinko and Lisper (2004) described seven categories of utterances associated with reflective listening that included: (1) *minimal encouragement,* (2) *direct encouragement,* (3) *reflecting fact,* (4) *reflecting emotion,* (5) *recapitulation,* (6) *open- and closed-ended questions on fact,* and (7) *questions on emotions.* These seven categories represent ways that clinicians can respond to clients that can enhance the therapeutic relationship and encourage them to go beyond the basic, problem-saturated descriptions that they initially provide. Lets take a look at each of these in more detail.

    1. *Minimal encouragement:* This involves short utterances such as "Uh-huh" or "Yes" or even head nodding that form part of the "active" participation that the listener uses to help the speaker to feel that the listener is engaged and interested. In addition to these verbal cues to the speaker that the listener is engaged, the listener should also "visibly tune in" (Egan, 2002) by maintaining appropriate eye contact, ensuring there are no physical barriers between the speaker and listener, keeping an open posture, and occasionally leaning in towards the speaker. Despite being in the background, these verbal and non-verbal actions by the listener can have a powerful effect on the feelings of engagement on the part of the speaker.

2. *Direct encouragement*: Students often think that they have to come up with a very insightful comment or question whenever the client comes to a stopping point in her or his story. This usually results in the student asking a "technical" question or moving on to a new topic rather than encouraging the client to continue with the story and build toward the thick descriptions that we are looking for. Instead of an insightful or even technical question or comment, the simple utterances related to explicit encouragement, such as "Go on," "Continue," or "Tell me more," will usually lead the client to dig deeper and start moving in the direction of more thick description. It is important for clinicians to understand that their role is to facilitate these thick descriptions and to let iMoments emerge rather than thinking that they need to make something happen.

3. & 4. *Reflecting fact and emotion*: Recall that Gordon's (1970) definition of reflective listening focuses on understanding the meaning and emotion of the speaker's message and reflecting it back to him or her in your own words for verification. This action is often referred to as "paraphrasing" and involves restating succinctly and tentatively what the speaker said. Paraphrases are always presented to the speaker *tentatively*—essentially as a question saying to the speaker, "This is what I heard; did I get it right?" By doing this, you are letting the listener know that you understand and, if you don't, that you are willing to be corrected. Again, this encourages the speaker to continue speaking, either expanding on or clarifying the story.

As implied by the two categories comprising this section, paraphrasing can occur at two levels, dealing with basic facts and events, and reflecting feelings and emotions related to those events. Although divided here into two separate categories, these rarely occur in isolation, so any paraphrasing that a listener does will almost always contain reflections of facts and reflections of emotions. The following example might be helpful to clarify this process of paraphrasing:

> **Parent:** *I don't understand why my son is not making any progress. It looks to me like all he ever does in therapy is play!*

> *Clinician: I can tell that you are frustrated by David's lack of progress and you don't feel that we are doing enough in the therapy sessions to help.*
>
> *Parent: Yes, I am just so anxious for him to start improving . . . and I just don't understand what playing games in these therapy sessions is doing for him.*
>
> *Clinician: It must be very difficult for you to watch him struggle with communicating the way he is and not be able to help him. Let me see if I can explain what we are trying to do and then we can talk about anything different that you think might be helpful. . . . You know him better than we do, so I'm really interested in your ideas.*

Here, the clinician reflected both facts and emotions to the parent, not only diffusing a difficult situation but recruiting the parent as an "expert" and helping address the feelings of helplessness reflected in the second part of the exchange.

5. *Recapitulation*: Also sometimes referred to as "summarizing," this involves focusing on the main points of the client's story to highlight them. It might be considered a "macro" version of the paraphrase—a tentative rewording of the important points from the entire session as opposed to specific utterances or stories for a paraphrase. Summaries will still focus on both facts and emotions, and are usually presented at the beginning and end of sessions. Beginning summaries are used to recall what happened at the last session—essentially setting the stage to pick up where you left off. Summaries at the end of sessions attempt to distill what happened over the length of a session into a few main points that the clients can take with them. As with paraphrasing, summaries are presented to the client in a tentative way, implying that you are open to changes as needed.

For example, Mary, an adolescent female who is coming to speech therapy for a vocal nodules, is just finishing a session in which she worked on practicing her less intense, breathy voice, reviewed her self-monitoring of her vocal rest and vocal hygiene, and discussed her reluctance to use her breathy voice around her friends. A summary that the clinician might present to Mary could be:

- *You are getting better at consistently producing the softer, breathier voice that we have been practicing.*
- *You are still struggling to achieve the vocal rest goals that we have set and you still get very irritated when you are on voice rest.*
- *You are being much more consistent with the vocal hygiene goals and seem to take pride in doing these activities to help your voice.*
- *You are feeling embarrassed and inhibited whenever you try to use your breathy voice around your friends and this is causing you to feel hopeless about being able to overcome your voice problem.*
- *Would you say this is accurate?*

6. & 7. *Open- and closed-ended questions on facts and emotions*: These different types of questions are used to get different types of information. Open-ended questions are questions that have no correct answer and require an explanation. They are designed to encourage a full, meaningful response, focusing on the speaker's own knowledge and feelings. Open-ended questions reflect the "client as expert" therapeutic stance that is part of our framework and demonstrate a respect of the client's knowledge, feelings, and opinions about his or her own problem. These types of questions frequently begin with words such as "Why," "What," and "How," or phrases such as "Tell me about . . ." and encourage the client to provide thick description.

In contrast, closed-ended questions are questions that are easily answered with a "Yes" or "No" response or a brief statement of information. These types of questions are designed to gather specific information, usually related to the "technical" aspects of the client's problem. Closed-ended questions serve an important function as part of the information-gathering process with a client. Difficulties arise, however, when clinicians ask closed-ended questions about topics that relate to the client's broader story. Table 9–1 shows some examples of closed-ended and open-ended questions

Table 9–1. Examples of Closed-Ended and Open-Ended Questions

Closed-Ended Question	Open-Ended Question
Has your stuttering changed since onset?	Tell me about your stuttering since its onset.
Have your hearing aids been working well?	Tell me about your experience wearing your hearing aids.
How many times were you able to successfully use your Vmax+ (AAC device) during your youth group meeting?	What was it like to use your Vmax+ during your youth group meeting?
Do you have trouble communicating with your husband since his stroke?	How are you communicating with your husband since his stroke? What has that been like for you?

focused on the same topic; consider the difference in the depth of information that you would receive from each type of question. Which types of questions encourage the client to provide thick descriptions?

Using Silence

People abhor silence the way nature abhors a vacuum. Novice and experienced clinicians alike will jump in at the slightest sign of any extended silence during a therapy session. Becoming comfortable with silence is a skill that is essential for encouraging thick descriptions for clients. This is especially true when working with clients with communication disorders, as they may sometimes take longer to formulate or express their thoughts. We have witnessed many beginning clinicians ask a question to, for example, a person who stutters and, due to the ensuing silence while the client is trying to respond, the clinicians get so uncomfortable that they just move on, asking another question or rephrasing the first question.

There is more to using silence, however, than simply giving clients time to respond. Silence is the primary vehicle for defining responsibility during the session (Luterman, 2001), and, given the client-centered and "client as expert" stance that make up our constructivist counseling framework, the responsibility for providing information and doing the hard work of adaptive change rests with the client. If, during an extended period of silence the clinician "rescues" the client, then she or he has taken over the responsibility for the session and cast him- or herself in the role of "fixing" the client's problem. Furthermore, extended silence gives clients time to think and reflect, and pushes clients to dig deeper, to examine previously ignored aspects of their story, and provide the thick descriptions that will be useful in identifying potential alternative stories.

During extended periods of silence, the clinician should maintain appropriate eye contact, with a look of expectation that suggests to the client that you are willing to wait as long as it takes and that you won't rescue them. As the therapeutic alliance between the client and clinician grows, periods of silence may get quite long but will be more comfortable, as both participants grow to appreciate the value of reflecting and don't perceive the silence as penalizing or judgmental.

Putting It All Together

Let's finish up by looking at a couple of examples that help illustrate how the type of listening we described in this chapter plays out in a clinical setting:

Mr. Brown

Mr. Brown is a 72-year-old individual who had been experiencing a gradual decline in hearing for over 12 years. He purchased binaural hearing aids approximately 9 years ago, but did not report much success with them, stating that he "rarely wears them." More recently, however, he has noticed that the quality of communication with his wife has declined and communication with others is almost non-existent as hc is in the habit of just deferring to his wife in communicative situations. In addition, he has begun to avoid using the telephone. He scheduled an appointment with Megan, an audiologist, at the encouragement of his wife, although he was full of doubts that his communication situation could improve.

Megan met with Mr. Brown for a hearing evaluation. After regular greetings and some brief discussion of the weather, Megan got started.

Megan: *So, Mr. Brown, tell me about what is happening with you.*

Mr. Brown: *Well, I have some trouble hearing sometimes. I got these hearing aids about 9 years ago but I never liked them much. They never were any good for me and they didn't really seem to make much difference. I can't hear anything, with or without them.*

Megan: *Well, that must be really frustrating . . . to have spent all that time and money and be getting no help from them!*

Mr. Brown: *You bet! I just don't think there is anything that is going to help . . . but Martha wanted me to come . . . so here we are!*

Megan: *Well, I can understand that you must be pretty discouraged. Maybe if we talk a little bit more about what you have been experiencing, we can come up with some ideas that might help?*

Silence. Mr. Brown thought for a while and Megan let him think.

Mr. Brown: *Well, I guess it couldn't hurt. What do you want to know?*

Megan: *Just tell me about yourself and what you like to do . . . and how the hearing loss has affected you.*

Mr. Brown: *Okay. I have always liked talking with people. Ask Martha . . . I'm a really friendly guy! She makes fun of me . . . says that I'll talk to anyone who will listen! But, I have to say, it's harder now than it used to be because I just find it hard to hear people a lot of the time . . . especially if it is a bit noisy!*

Megan: *I imagine that is difficult for you—not being able to do something that you enjoy?*

Mr. Brown: *It makes me a bit sad sometimes when I stop myself from going up to someone but I still talk to people . . . just maybe not as much as I used to.*

Megan: *Can you tell me more about how the hearing loss is getting in the way of things you like to do?*

Mr. Brown: *Church has been a real problem! I quit going for a while but now Martha and I go to the early service. It is small and they don't play the organ. I can hear the preacher better but we kind of miss the full service sometimes . . . and we don't get to sit with our friends like we used to.*

Megan: *It sounds like that is something that you really miss?*

Mr. Brown: *Yes, I think we really do miss it. I sure wish I wasn't such a broken down old man! I'm the one stopping us from going!*

Megan: *You sound really frustrated by not being able to go to the service that you want to . . . maybe even a bit angry?*

Mr. Brown: *Maybe . . . I just feel bad for Martha.*

Megan: *Uh-huh. It really seems like this hearing loss has taken some things away from you that were important to you? Is that accurate?*

Mr. Brown: *Yes, I would say so.*

Megan: *Tell me about some of the things you have done to try to resist the influence of the hearing loss.*

Mr. Brown: *Well, I got these hearing aids about 9 years ago.*

Megan: *Uh-huh. You showed them to me before. Tell me about them.*

Mr. Brown: *They helped some at first, with the TV, and in quiet places, but not all the time . . . and I didn't like the way they sounded . . . and they weren't very comfortable. So, I don't wear them much anymore.*

Megan let Mr. Brown sit in silence for a while as he seemed to be thinking. . . .

Mr. Brown: *I also tried watching people's faces more. I noticed that I missed more of a conversation when people turned their back on me. Martha used to do that, sometimes she still does, but I tell her, "You have to look at me when you talk!" She's getting better, but I still have to remind her occasionally.*

Megan: *Uh-huh. That is a great strategy . . . and it sounds like it has helped some?*

Mr. Brown: *Yeah, it has . . . but not really a whole lot. I also tried just telling people to speak up! You know, not trying to hide that I couldn't hear too well. That works okay sometimes but kind of makes me feel like I'm just giving up...and maybe I am! I just don't see anything that is going to really help!*

Megan: *Thank you for sharing that, Mr. Brown. I really appreciate you being so open with me! From what I heard you say, it seems that you've been pretty active in trying to find ways to resist the influence of the hearing problem?*

Mr. Brown: *Hmm . . . I guess you could say that. But everything has just been avoiding the truth!*

Megan: *Well, that might be one way to look at it. Another way might be to see what you have been doing as very resourceful. You have done a lot to find ways to challenge the impact that the hearing loss has been having on your life.*

Mr. Brown: *Well . . . I've never really thought of it that way. . . . You could be right. I usually do seem to find a way to get around problems, even if sometimes it doesn't seem like a very good solution. Martha has always said that I was a good problem-solver!*

Megan: *There you go . . . a problem-solver! I wonder if we can work together to find even more resources that might be helpful in solving this hearing loss problem?*

Megan then proceeded with standard audiological testing and discussed the findings with Mr. Brown. Megan identified hearing aids that would be a good choice for Mr. Brown's loss and should provide improved performance and fit compared to his previous aids. Rather than presenting the idea of amplification as a "solution," however, Megan suggested to Mr. Brown that new hearing aids might be *one resource* that he could recruit to help him "problem-solve" the hearing loss. Megan also discussed several other "resources" that Mr. Brown could use in his attempts at problem solving. He agreed to try the treatment plan that Megan proposed, which included new hearing aids, as well as various communication strategy sessions and learning about hearing assistance technology.

Mark

Mark was a 22-year-old man who stuttered. He had been working on smoothing and controlling his stuttering for many years and was getting quite good at it. He was experiencing a period of relatively easy and consistent control over his disfluencies, a period that had been going for approximately 4 months, when we met after he had spent some time working at a school. On this day, Mark was clearly not happy and wanted to talk rather than jump into our regular (technical) "stuttering treatment" activities.

> AD: *So, Mark, it looks to me like there is something on your mind. Do you want to talk about it?*
>
> Mark: *Yeah. It hasn't been a good week! It was mainly this one experience . . . but it has really messed with my head!*
>
> Silence . . .
>
> Mark: *I had an IEP meeting the other day with some parents, teachers, and the principal all there . . . and I totally lost it!*
>
> AD: *Lost it? What do you mean?*
>
> Mark: *Well, I was SO disfluent! I couldn't control anything. It was the most I have stuttered in a long time!*

AD: *Okay. Well, that must have been tough. It sounds like it really hit you hard.*

Mark: *Yeah. It was hard. I was embarrassed and just mad at myself! I mean, I've been doing so well now for a pretty long time. So it kind of surprised me that I couldn't control it, you know? I have really been in control lately and even in difficult situations, I have been able to keep control. But this meeting . . . was just a disaster!*

AD: *Wow. It sounds like it really disappointed you . . . that you couldn't get control of the stuttering?*

Mark: *Yeah. It really was disappointing. I got through the meeting but it just made me realize that I need to practice more . . . do more work on using my controls.*

AD: *You mentioned that "it kind of surprised you" that you couldn't control the stuttering in this meeting. I'm interested in what you meant. Could you tell me more about that?*

Mark: *Well, it just surprised me because I had been doing so well. You know, I had been able to control my stuttering pretty much all the time while at school, and most of the time at other times as well. It has been a long time since I struggled like that. So, yeah, it did surprise me.*

AD: *That's really interesting. I wonder if that tells you anything about how you are changing?*

Mark: *I don't know. It tells me that I need to practice more!*

AD: *Hmm. Maybe, but does it tell you anything about YOU and how YOU are changing?*

Some extended silence as Mark contemplates the question and his response. . . .

Mark: *Well, I guess it shows me that I have been doing well . . . and that I shouldn't take it for granted. Is that what you are looking for?*

AD: *Ha! I am not necessarily looking for anything! But I am trying to get you to think about how you might view this experience in an alternative way. So far, you have interpreted it as indicating that you need to practice your "technical" skills more. How might the fact that you were surprised by the stuttering tell you something about how you are changing in your thinking?*

Again, some extended silence (this time longer than before) as Mark contemplates the question and his response. . . .

Mark: *Okay, I think I know where you are going with this! Because I was surprised by the stuttering . . . it means that I wasn't expecting to stutter . . . which is a big change from what I would have expected before. Yeah, I see that. Hmm. That is kind of interesting!*

AD: *It is, isn't it? From what I have seen, a stutterer always expects to stutter and is never surprised by it!*

Mark: *That's true. I always knew that stuttering would be there. . . . Even if I was having a good day, I always knew the stuttering would be there if I hit a tough situation or word. You're right. . . . I was never surprised by it before!*

AD: *Hmm. So, what does that say to you about how you are changing?*

More silence. I could see the turmoil in Mark's face as he wrestled with the conclusion that he was coming to but just couldn't bring himself to accept, as it was in conflict of his long-held core construct of himself as a "stutterer". . . .

Mark: *Well, I guess it says that I am not...well, not really a stutterer? Or, at least, becoming not a stutterer?*

I let Mark's question hang out there for a while. We both sat there and looked at each other.

AD: *You sound a little unsure about that statement. What are you feeling right now?*

Mark: *I don't know. It is a little hard to believe. But, at the same time, I really WAS surprised that I couldn't control my stuttering . . . so I wasn't expecting to stutter . . . (nodding his head) . . . I wasn't expecting to stutter. Hmm. That's pretty cool!*

This was a profound conversation for Mark. We revisited this alternative story many times in subsequent conversations and, according to Mark, it formed a foundation from which he has continued to build.

Conclusions

Reflective or therapeutic listening is a major component of effective counseling. It is a natural extension of the person-centered therapeutic stance that is a central aspect of our framework—that the client is the expert about his or her own problem—and is the clinician's primary tool in encouraging the thick descriptions that are needed for clients and clinicians to encounter the clues (iMoments) to alternative narratives that may lead to preferred identities.

References

Egan, G. (2002). *The skilled helper: A problem-management and opportunity development approach to helping* (7th ed.). Pacific Grove, CA: Brooks/Cole.

Gordon, T. (1970). *PET: Parent effectiveness training.* New York, NY: Wyden.

Luterman, D. M. (2001). *Counseling persons with communication disorders and their families.* (4th ed.). Austin, TX: Pro-Ed, Inc.

Rautalinko, E., & Lisper, H. O. (2004). Effects of training reflective listening in a corporate setting. *Journal of Business and Psychology, 18,* 281–299.

Rogers, C. R. (1961). *On becoming a person.* Boston, MA: Houghton Mifflin.

Rogers, C. R. (1980). *A way of being.* Boston, MA: Houghton Mifflin.

10

FACILITATING RECONSTRUCTION

In this chapter, we look more closely at some of the tools available to the clinician to aid in the reconstruction process. In Clinician's Toolbox #3 in Chapter 8, we introduced the concept of *externalizing* as a way that clinicians can engage clients in conversations that separate the problem from the person. In this chapter we expand on this and provide examples of some of the types of questions that might encourage clients to consider alternative constructions of their problem.

Also in Chapter 8, we introduced the concept of *iMoments*— those taken-for-granted, usually ignored experiences that reflect some form of resistance to the dominant problem narrative. In this chapter, we explore further the different types of iMoments that might be found in clients' thick descriptions of their lives and we look at questions that clinicians can use to elicit or expand such iMoments.

In Chapter 2 we presented the case of Flora and how she was able to overcome fear and anxiety related to her swallowing problem by experimenting with new behaviors and ways of construing events. In this chapter, we revisit this concept of *experimenting with experience* and look at how this fits neatly into activities and processes that clinicians are already engaged in with their clients.

Finally, in Chapter 8 we briefly discussed *co-construction* as one of the foundational aspects of our counseling framework. In this chapter, we look more deeply at how clinicians can employ outsider witnesses to help their clients elaborate their emerging preferred stories.

Externalizing

The description of externalizing provided in Chapter 8 highlighted the use of a word or short phrase to "name" the problem, thereby creating opportunities for the client and clinician to engage in "externalizing conversations" that can help change the way that the client thinks about the problem. To explain this further, let's look at this idea of naming the problem in more detail.

In this context, "naming the problem" is done to *objectify* or *personify* the problem being experienced as oppressive, making it a *separate entity* and thus external to the person (White & Epston, 1990). In this way, externalizing language can be useful in encouraging persons to move from feeling like a "problem person" to being a "person with a problem." Referring to the problem as an external "entity," using comments like "What did *Hearing Loss* say to you to make you avoid that party?" or "*Stuttering* seemed to be pushing you around yesterday," can help in recruiting the person to be an active participant in the treatment process, rather than feeling like a problem person who requires "fixing" by the clinician. As such, externalizing language places the client at odds with the problem, essentially teaming the client with the clinician to resist the problem's influence on his or her life and relationships.

The concepts of externalizing can be difficult for some clients to grasp or they might feel inhibited talking about their problem as an entity. A number of the tools in Part IV of this book have been designed to promote and strengthen an externalizing of the problem and may help clients get a clearer understanding of this concept. (See Chapter 15: *Autobiography of the Problem*; Chapter 17: *Drawing*; Chapter 18: *Dear John Letter*; and Chapter 22: *Chair Work*.)

iMoments

For some clients, the insights that they develop through naming their problem can be extremely therapeutic. They can change their attitude toward the problem, taking a stance and pushing back against the problem's influence. For most, however, the process of change is more difficult and requires additional facilitation from the clinician. As discussed previously, thick descriptions and externalizing can help clients begin to view and talk about their problem in a different way. Often, exploration of these different ways of thinking about the problem can lead to the identification of *iMoments*—those taken-for-granted times when the client resisted or overcame the effects of the problem—providing a window into a potential alternative story and preferred identity.

As indicated in Chapter 8, Gonçalves and colleagues (e.g., Gonçalves et al., 2012; Gonçalves & Ribeiro, 2012; Gonçalves et al., 2010) identified five types of iMoments that may occur in client's discourse and which have been associated with successful therapy.

Protest iMoments involve some form of resistance against the problem, mustering energy to oppose its influence in the client's life. For example, a client who declares that she is "sick and tired" of the hoarseness caused by her overuse of her voice through speaking loudly is showing protest in this sense, and signaling a readiness to experiment with new ways of speaking.

Reflection iMoments entail new understandings or thoughts about the client or the problem that depart from the plot of the dominant narrative. An illustration of this might be a man with stuttering who recognizes that as uncomfortable as his disfluency makes him feel in work situations at his desk job, it also protects him from pursuing a potentially more satisfying but anxiety-producing career in sales.

Action iMoments refer to specific behaviors that challenge the dominance of the problematic narrative. For instance, a typically quiet student with an articulation problem who speaks up in class would be displaying this form of change, inviting the clinician's attention to other new behaviors that signal hope and courage to make more of an appearance in her life.

Reconceptualization iMoments involve meta-reflection on the process of change, demonstrating that a client not only recognizes that he or she has changed, but also can describe the process by which this occurred. An example would be a client who acknowledges a new sense of pride in achieving more control over his fluency through hard work and practice of skills, and recognizes that this reflects the same "stick-to-it-iveness" that has served him well in dealing with other challenges. Reconceptualization implies seeing the difference between the past and the present, and the bridge that allowed the client to transition from one to the other.

Performing change iMoments refer to the generalization of change, or to anticipating new experiences, projects, or activities. For instance, a man with hearing impairment who overcomes his initial reluctance to consult an audiologist, who is fitted with a hearing aid, and who begins to use it not only at home but also in a range of social situations he has long avoided would be performing change in this sense. The client may describe this form of iMoment in a few sentences, but unlike action iMoments, performing change involves modifying behavior across a longer period of time and usually in several situations.

In Chapter 8 we discussed how to use these iMoments to help clients begin to re-author their personal narratives by asking them to elaborate them and encouraging them to explore these alternative stories and preferred identities.

Relative Influence Questions

White and Epston (1990) suggest that many clients may benefit from additional help to externalize their problem and identify iMoments. They suggest using *"relative influence questioning"* as a way to effectively assist persons to externalize the problem and explore possible alternative storylines. Relative influence questions are divided into two categories, "mapping the influence of the problem in the life and relationships of the person" and "mapping the influence of the person and their relationships in the life of the problem." The first category includes questions that encourage the person to become aware of, and to describe, the problem's sphere of influence, and to identify the effect of the problem across various facets of the person's life and relationships. This is the goal of the "thick descriptions" discussed previously in Chapters 8 and 9.

The second category includes questions that relate to opening up a new way for the person to view the problem. These questions encourage the person to acknowledge and identify, often for the first time, that he or she has an influence on the life of the problem. These questions often generate information that contradicts the problem-saturated description of the person's life and can assist in identifying his or her competence and resourcefulness (i.e., iMoments).

Epston and White (1999) suggest a series of relative influence-type questions designed to help clinicians facilitate the process of change in psychotherapy. DiLollo, Neimeyer, and Manning (2002) adapted these questions for use with persons who stutter. The questions presented here are further adapted to be applicable to clients with any communication or swallowing disorder.

Unique Outcome Questions

These questions are designed to invite clients to acknowledge actions and intentions that contradict the dominant story—the "unique outcomes," as Epston and White refer to them, or "iMoments," as we described them back in Chapter 8. Examples of these types of questions include:

- "Have there been other times when you have been able to overcome *The Problem's* hold over your speech? How did you feel when this happened?"
- "Can you imagine a time in the future in which you might resist or overcome *The Problem's* influence over your speech? Over your life in general?"

Clients responding to such questions might begin to "notice" more clearly the times and ways that they "hold their own" against the attention-getting "demands" of *The Problem*, and think about how they might expand their influence over the problem in future situations. By showing clear interest in the easily missed details of these accounts, clinicians can help "grow the story" of the client's competence, which is further supported through the inquiry strategies outlined below.

Unique Account Questions

The goal of these questions is to facilitate development of a preferred alternative story centered on previously identified unique outcomes. Unique account questions invite clients to make sense of exceptions to the dominant narrative that may not have even registered previously as significant and to retain them as part of an emerging coherent narrative. These questions also serve to "historicize" the development of solutions to the client's problem, grounding them in the client's pre-existing strengths. In this way, the client develops a greater sense of ownership of the solutions, which provides him or her with the capacity to redeploy them at some time in the future should similar challenges arise (Epston & White, 1999). These types of questions might include:

- "Given how familiar *The Problem* is to you, how were you able to protest its pushing you around?"
- "How might you stand up to *The Problem* in the future and refuse its requirements of you?"
- "What can you tell me about your history that would help me understand the development of your ability to defeat *The Problem*?"

The clinician can then respond by prompting the client to consider past and present strengths (e.g., persistence, resilience, ingenuity) that contributed to these preferred outcomes. In so doing, the client and clinician in effect work together to construct an alternative story of the client's identity, one that is less problem "saturated."

Unique Redescription Questions

These questions aim to help clients reflect on, and develop meaning from, the unique accounts that they have identified. As they redescribe themselves, the clinician can direct their attention to the conclusions and realizations reached about their capabilities and competencies. These questions further "historicize" the identified unique accounts, helping clients to recognize this new self-knowledge as a reflection of long established personal and relationship strengths and resources.

A further importance of historicizing a re-description of self for persons with communication and swallowing disorders is to provide a sense that this is not a "new" self, but a part that has always been present. These types of questions might include:

- "What does this achievement reflect about the sort of person you are that is important for you to know? Are you the first to know this about yourself, or have others known this about you in the past? If others have known this, what told them?"

Prompted by such questions, clients tend to glimpse, often for the first time, the outline of a broader identity beyond the problem, one that encompasses valued characteristics and competencies that were previously eclipsed by the story of *The Problem*. Clinicians can help call up these new perspectives by presenting clients with a series of successes and asking, "What do all of these accomplishments tell us about the kind of person you are, about the dependable strengths that you might carry with you into the future?" The preferred story of self can be further consolidated by sharing with the client change-affirming progress notes (Neimeyer, 1993) or other therapeutic documents (see Chapter 24).

Unique Possibility Questions

These questions invite clients to speculate about various personal and relational alternatives that derive from their unique accounts and redescriptions. They are designed to promote discussion of such alternative possibilities as well as specific steps that might be taken to realize them. They are generally framed as "future-oriented, backward-looking" questions, which ask clients to imagine themselves arriving at some valued personal or relational destination and then to look back to the present time and determine which steps they are currently taking are most important to reaching that destination and what subsequent steps would be most helpful in achieving that goal (Epston & White, 1999).

Such questions might include:

- "What will the future be like without *The Problem's* influence dominating your life? How is this future different from the one that *The Problem* would have planned for you?"
- "Knowing what you now know about yourself and your preference for living life without *The Problem's* influence, how will this knowledge affect your next step?"

In an ironic sense, successful therapy for long-term communication disorders can engender anxiety, precisely because it disrupts the continuity of the client's self-narrative, albeit in desirable directions (Neimeyer, 2000). Unique possibility questions mitigate this disruption by helping the person envision a preferred future that is coherent with the best moments of the past, rather than at odds with its essential meaning. For instance, a client might respond to the above questions by conjuring a future characterized by greater self-worth and intimacy with others, qualities that are already foreshadowed in recent steps that the client has taken to assert himself or herself in social relationships. By encouraging the client to outline this preferred future in as much detail as possible, the clinician encourages the client to construct a more tangible and less threatening image toward which to move.

Unique Circulation Questions

Personal narratives are constructed and lived out in social contexts (Drewery & Winslade, 1997; Neimeyer, 2000), and the construction and anchoring of any new personal narratives must also be performed in a social context. White and Epston (1990) state that the inclusion of others in the newly developing story is essential to anchoring and continuing the development of that narrative.

Examples of these questions might be:

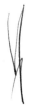

- "Now that you have overcome *The Problem's* influence in your life, who else should know about it? What difference do you think it would make to their attitude toward you if they knew this news?"
- "Of the significant people in your life, who do you anticipate would have difficulty accepting the new life you have chosen, free from *The Problem's* influence?"

For example, a fluency client might answer such questions as these by noting the pleasant surprise and acceptance shown by certain friends exposed to his newfound fluency, a fact that could be elaborated upon in response to further clinician questions about their favorable attitudes. Alternatively, the clinician might enlarge the audience for the performance of the new self by helping identify specific persons or groups (perhaps relatives living far away who might be given a phone call) who would also notice and reinforce the "fluent self" role. Such questioning strategies further strengthen the new identity by anchoring it in the positive appraisals of others.

Questions That Historicize Unique Outcomes

These questions serve to develop the emerging story, establish it as having a memorable history, and increase the likelihood of it being carried forward into the future. These types of questions might include, for example:

- "Of the people who knew you growing up, who would have been most likely to predict that you would break free from *The Problem's* influence?"
- "What qualities would this person have seen in you that would have led him/her to believe that you would have been able to achieve what you have?"

By combining aspects of audience recruitment and "temporal weaving," tacking back and forth between past promise and present possibilities, inquiries like these further enhance the meaning of the emerging self-image, laying the foundation for a different and more hopeful autobiography. Clinicians in a sense serve as co-editors of the emerging self-narrative, assisting the client as author to develop a credible character capable of playing a different role on the social stage (Neimeyer, 2000).

Experimenting with Experience

Externalizing the problem and identifying iMoments can be helpful to many clients in starting the process of changing their self-narrative from one dominated by the effects of the problem to a more functional and preferred story. As clients begins to recognize potential new ways of thinking and acting, there is potential for difficulties to arise as they may find that acting in ways that are different from their long-established core role constructs comes with feelings of anxiety, fear, and even guilt. Recall the discussion in Chapter 5 regarding constructs and emotions and the research from Chapter 7 suggesting that persons who stutter, for example, have a difficult time transitioning to a "fluent speaker role" and frequently relapse back to their more familiar and safe "stutterer role."

In Chapter 5 we also introduced Kelly's (1955/1991) concept of the "experience cycle" as the process by which the construct system refines constructs, testing the validity of old constructs and updating them if they do not provide accurate anticipation. When functioning optimally, the experience cycle consists of five phases that include *anticipation, investment, encounter with the event, assessment of anticipation,* and *revision of construing* (Butler, 2009).

Sometimes, however, this process fails to eliminate constructs that are not providing adequate predictions, usually because they are strongly held "core" constructs or constructs related to an area of difficulty or conflict. In such cases, clients need help to revise these constructs and replace them with preferred, more functional constructs. The case of Flora, described in Chapter 2, is an example of the experience cycle not revising a construct related to an area of discomfort. In her case, Flora was unable to revise her constructs about eating in front of family members because she was unwilling or unable to test her constructs about what might occur. In such cases, just talking about change is not enough to overcome the strength of the constructs (Neimeyer, 2009). The example described at the start of Chapter 2 regarding anxiety about flying clearly demonstrated this principle, as none of the talking about the relative safety of flying and related statistics had any impact on the constructs underlying the fear.

In these circumstances, when clients are clinging to constructs that need to be revised, clinicians can facilitate the "experience cycle" by engaging clients in experimenting with experience (Epting, Gemignani, & Cross, 2005). This process involves deciding on a construct or set of constructs to address in an experiment to be performed in the outside world (i.e., outside the therapy room). For clients with communication disorders, these will often be constructs that relate to how they will be perceived when enacting new or different ways of communicating, such as speaking fluently for a PWS, using a voice of a different pitch or intensity, using an AAC device, producing certain sounds differently, or wearing hearing aids. One of the aspects that makes this such a useful tool for speech-language pathologists in particular, but also for audiologists in rehabilitation settings, is that the experiments at the core of this process are typically the same as the homework assignments frequently given to clients to practice their emerging speech or language skills outside of the therapy room. Consequently, this is something that clinicians are already having clients do; it is the preparations for the experiment and the debriefing following the experiment that are different, if the clinician is working from our constructivist framework.

Prior to embarking on the experiment, the client is invited to describe both positive and negative predictions of what will happen, how she or he will feel, and how others involved will react. Typically, these predictions are recorded so that they can be reviewed after the experiment is completed. Sometimes clients find it useful to role-play the experiment in the therapy room with the clinician before carrying out the experiment in public. Once the experiment has been completed, the clinician must invest time into debriefing, as this is when the revision of the constructs begins.

Typically, speech-language pathologists review homework assignments by checking on how successful the client was in executing the target behavior. Working within our constructivist framework, however, means that clinicians recognize that the homework (or experiment) is about more than behavior change. By reviewing with the client how things went during the experiment—how she or he felt and how others reacted—and then comparing what happened with what the client predicted would happen (i.e., his or her existing constructs), the clinician is essentially facilitating an "experience cycle" that can start the process of changing constructs that are invalidated by the client's experiences. Usually, multiple experiments are required to begin to impact strongly held constructs.

Consider the example of Tim, a 7-year-old boy who is receiving articulation therapy to correct some speech-sound errors. *Tim is performing very well in the therapy room, consistently hitting 90% or better for his target sounds in both sentences and in conversation. His teacher, however, reports that Tim is not making any progress in class and another teacher reports that Tim is not using his improved sounds when on the playground. To many clinicians, this would be seen as a problem with "generalization" and compliance, with the answer being to assign Tim some homework assignments to practice his sounds away from the therapy room. Working within the constructivist framework, however, the clinician might suspect that there is more to Tim's story than just non-compliance. After the clinician invites Tim to talk about how he is using his new sounds away from therapy, Tim reveals that he is afraid to use his sounds in front of his friends because they will laugh and make fun of him, as they already tease him about going to speech therapy. In response to this, the clinician sets up a series of experiments for Tim to try. Framing them as experiments and working with Tim to start with a setting that is the least intimidating encourages Tim to take these on rather than just keep avoiding them. The clinician starts out by asking Tim to describe what he thinks is going to happen when he uses his sounds in the classroom (the environment chosen by Tim as the least intimidating). The clinician records Tim's predictions (i.e., his current constructs) that kids will laugh and he will be embarrassed. Tim engages in the experiment before the next therapy session, being sure to pay attention to how he felt and how others reacted. At the next speech therapy session, the clinician asks Tim how things went. The focus is on his feelings and the reactions of others, although the clinician is still interested in how well he was able to hit his speech targets. As Tim talks about how no one seemed to even notice when he used his sounds and that he was not embarrassed, the clinician weaves into the conversation Tim's predictions and helps him see how they were not validated. Of course, it is likely that Tim will protect his beliefs about how others will react, possibly by pointing out that "This was just one time. Maybe they just weren't paying attention" or "Well, it didn't happen in the class because the teacher was there but it will happen in the playground." It may take multiple experiments before Tim starts to change his constructs and feels comfortable enacting the behavior changes learned in the therapy room.*

Selling the Story

One of the foundational aspects of our constructivist framework is the personal narrative. In Chapter 6 and again in Chapter 8, we have described how we make sense of life through the "storying" of lived experience (Madigan & Goldner, 1998) and that these stories, or personal narratives, not only reflect but also influence how we see the world. It is not only the stories that we tell about ourselves, however, that form our personal narrative, but also the stories that others tell about us, or, as Winslade and Monk (1999) stated, "We are not the sole authors of our stories" (p. 3). This concept of the social construction of our personal narratives, therefore, plays an important role in helping clients with communication disorders establish preferred identities related to themselves as communicators. Consequently, another fundamental aspect of our constructivist counseling framework is the concept of co-construction (see Chapter 8).

Outsider-witness practices (White, 1995, 2007) are one way that narrative therapists facilitate the co-construction of preferred identities with their clients. Although this formal procedure, sometimes also referred to as "definitional ceremonies," has been used effectively with clients with communication disorders (Leahy et al., 2012; Logan, 2007), most speech-language pathologists and audiologists will likely not engage in these types of practices due to time and facility constraints. This does not mean, however, that this aspect of the framework should be ignored. It is important for clients to "sell" their story to significant others in their lives and to have their story retold by various outsiders that might include family members but also other clinicians or even other clients. Typically, as a preferred story of resistance to the problem emerges, clinicians will be the first line of retelling as they reflect back to the client various aspects of the story and what it means to the client. As the story continues to build, the clinician may invite other "witnesses" into the therapy room (with the client's consent, of course) to engage in a discussion of the changes that the client is making. As mentioned before, these outsiders might include other clinicians, other clients, family members, or friends. It is important to engage family members and significant people from the client's environment in this aspect of treatment as they will need to support the preferred story (by accepting it and continuing to re-tell it) when the client is ready to fully integrate it into his or her life. Consider this clinical anecdote: *A man had just completed a two-week intensive, residential fluency training program in which he achieved increased fluency and worked on assertiveness and self confidence. A week after his return home, the speech-language pathologist in charge of the program received a call from the man's irate wife, complaining that her husband had changed and he was no longer the man she married!* Clearly, some inclusion of the wife in the telling and re-telling of her husband's preferred story may have averted this potentially disastrous situation.

Conclusions

In this chapter we expanded on the concepts introduced in Chapter 8 as part of the constructivist counseling framework. Although there is a significant amount of detail in this chapter that, at first glance, may appear daunting and confusing to speech-language pathologists and audiologists not trained specifically as counselors, we remind readers that these details are presented to enhance your background knowledge and understanding—NOT as a prescriptive method of counseling.

In summary, this chapter outlined ways for clinicians to facilitate reconstruction of the client's personal narrative through *externalizing, identifying iMoments, using relative influence questions, experimenting with experience,* and *selling the story.* Experienced clinicians tend to weave back and forth among these processes in a natural flow that reflects the needs and preferences of the client. What might this look like in the actual give-and-take between clinician and client? One answer to this question appears in the chapter to follow, which offers an extended consideration of constructivist counseling with a person who stutters and draws on each of these practices in an organic way to foster reconstruction, not only of the client's patterns of speech, but also of his sense of himself.

References

Butler, R. (2009). Encounters of the puzzling kind: The organizational corollary in relation to self-construing. In R. Butler (Ed.), *Reflections in personal construct theory* (pp. 111–129). London, UK: Wiley-Blackwell.

DiLollo, A., Neimeyer, R. A., & Manning, W. H. (2002). A personal construct psychology view of relapse: Indications for a narrative therapy component to stuttering treatment. *Journal of Fluency Disorders, 27,* 19–42.

Drewery, W., & Winslade, J. (1997). The theoretical story of narrative therapy. In G. Monk, J. Winslade, K. Crocket, & D. Epston (Eds.), *Narrative therapy in practice: The archaeology of hope.* San Francisco, CA: Jossey-Bass Publishers.

Epston, D., & White, M. (1999). Termination as a right of passage: Questioning strategies for a therapy of inclusion. In R. A. Neimeyer & R. J. Mahoney (Eds.), *Constructivism in psychotherapy.* Washington, DC: American Psychological Association.

Epting, F. R., Gemignani, M., & Cross, M. C. (2005). An audacious adventure: Personal construct counseling and psychotherapy. In F. Fransella (Ed.), *The essential practitioner's handbook of personal construct psychology* (pp. 113–121). West Sussex, UK: John Wiley & Sons.

Gonçalves, M. M., Mendes, I., Cruz, G., Ribeiro, A., Angus, L., & Greenberg, L. (2012). Innovative moments and change in client-centered therapy. *Psychotherapy Research.* doi: 10.1080=10503307.2012.662605

Gonçalves, M. M., & Ribeiro, A. P. (2012). Therapeutic change, innovative moments, and the reconceptualization of the self: A dialogical account. *International Journal for Dialogical Science, 6,* 81-98.

Gonçalves, M. M., Santos, A., Matos, M., Salgado, J., Mendes, J., Ribeiro, A., . . . Gonçalves, J. (2010). Innovations in psychotherapy: Tracking the narrative construction of change. In J. D. Raskin, S. K. Bridges, & R. A. Neimeyer (Eds.), *Studies in meaning 4: Constructivist perspectives on theory, practice, and social justice.* New York, NY: Pace University Press.

Kelly, G. A. (1955/1991). *The psychology of personal constructs.* New York, NY: Routledge.

Leahy, M. M., O'Dwyer, M., & Ryan, F. (2012). Witnessing stories: Definitional ceremonies in narrative therapy with adults who stutter. *Journal of Fluency Disorders, 37*(4), 234-241. doi:10.1016/j.jfludis.2012.03.001

Logan, J. (2007). From client to consultant: Developing "outsider-witness practices" with adults who stammer. In J. Au-Yeung & M. M. Leahy (Eds.), *Research, treatment and self-help in fluency disorders: New horizons. Proceedings of the 5th world congress on fluency disorders* (pp. 325-332). Dublin, Ireland: International Fluency Association.

Madigan, S. P., & Goldner, E. M. (1998). A narrative approach to anorexia. In M. F. Hoyt (Ed.), *The handbook of constructive therapies: Innovative approaches from leading practitioners.* San Francisco, CA: Jossey-Bass Publishers.

Neimeyer, R. A. (1993). Constructivist approaches to the measurement of meaning. In G. J. Neimeyer (Ed.), *Constructivist assessment: A casebook* (pp. 58-103). Newbury Park: CA: Sage.

Neimeyer, R. A. (2000). Narrative disruptions in the construction of self. In R. A. Neimeyer & J. D. Raskin (Eds.), *Constructions of disorder: Meaning making frameworks for psychotherapy* (pp. 207-241). Washington, DC: American Psychological Association.

Neimeyer, R. A. (2009). *Constructivist psychotherapy.* London, UK & New York, NY: Routledge.

White, M. (1995). *Re-authoring lives: Interviews and essays.* Adelaide, Australia: Dulwich Centre Publications.

White, M. (2007). *Maps of narrative practice.* New York, NY: Norton.

White, M., & Epston, D. (1990). *Narrative means to therapeutic ends.* New York, NY: Norton.

Winslade, J. & Monk, G. (1999). *Narrative counseling in schools: Powerful and brief.* Thousand Oaks, CA: Corwin Press.

11

EXTERNALIZATION AND RELATIVE INFLUENCE QUESTIONING: A CASE ILLUSTRATION

What makes for a good story? According to literary theorists, narratives really become compelling when they feature a protagonist or main character who is pursuing some form of goal or objective, and who meets with obstacles, often in the form of an antagonist whose opposition or challenge needs to be overcome for the story to reach a satisfying conclusion (Neimeyer, 2000). Something in us is drawn to formulate experience in these terms, whether the resulting tale takes the form of a comedy, adventure, detective story, or heroic epic. In fact, one might even say that the difficulty of formulating "psychological problems" in these terms—as when we as would-be agents of change seem to be the same ones who block our own progress—is what makes such problems so intractable. How can we find a way forward beyond our problems when we are the very ones responsible for them? Faced with this blurring of person and problem (which is too often reinforced by a social world that blames us for our difficulty), we easily get muddled and discouraged, and aren't sure where to turn . . . except toward greater self-blame, and in the case of many communication disorders, self-isolation as well.

It is here, as we noted in the previous chapter, that narrative therapy could offer some helpful tools. One of these is *externalization*, that is, separating the person from the problem in a way that clarifies their relationship to each other. The second and related tool is *relative influence questioning*, in effect examining the history of the problem's influence on the person of the client, and the person's influence on the problem. This "give and take" between the client and problem typically varies widely across different circumstances. A client who is challenged with partial deafness might find that some activities in his life, like attending a symphony, are particularly dominated by his hearing problem, as some interludes are almost too soft to hear or appreciate, and others are piercing and painful. At other times, he might feel more agency in "pushing back" against the problem: when dining out with others, assertively selecting a chair at a table that maximizes his ability to hear the high-pitched voice of one of his dining companions. And at still other times—as when reading quietly at night—his hearing might not be much of a factor one way or another, except for the cresting and falling of the tinnitus that has become a near constant companion. It can therefore be illuminating for clinician and client to examine closely the interaction between the person and the problem, especially as intervention of many kinds is designed to help clients get more of an "upper hand" in relation to a difficulty or disorder that too often has left them feeling helpless. As we will see, the constructivist ideas of the experience cycle and experimenting with experience are natural companions in this effort.

Talking Back to Stuttering

To illustrate the use of these narrative and constructivist processes, we'll consider three excerpts from Bob's counseling with Walt, a mature businessman who is presently taking some executive training classes. Walt has stuttered for as long as he can remember, and initially was skeptical that another round of speech therapy could help him with the social problems that were beginning to limit not only his personal life, but also his career trajectory. Walt had sought conventional behavioral therapies to modify his speech in the past, with some positive effect, but which ultimately proved short-lived.

A Narrative Beginning

Interspersed with refreshers on these skills and encouragement to do "field experiments" with them in social contexts, therapy also took a narrative turn in order to clarify stuttering's influence on Walt's sense of himself, and then to help him find more "voice" in the relationship. An early session began:

> **Bob:** Well Walt, it's good to meet with you again this week, and to have a chance to follow up some of our previous conversations about how your speech has been going and your contact with people. (*Walt looks at the floor.*) You kind of glanced down at that. What, what comes to you as I ask that question?
>
> **Walt:** Well I think m-m-m-m- my speech is about the same since we met. I'm, actually I may . . . I may even be stuttering more.
>
> **Bob:** Uh huh, yeah.
>
> **Walt:** So I, uh, I guess I would say it has been a. . . . been a- been a hard week with p-p-people.
>
> **Bob:** This has been a week in the presence of other people. You spent quite a lot of time socially as we had talked about?
>
> **Walt:** Well, not as m—not as much as I wanted to. Not as much as I said I was, um, going to. I didn't participate in class at all, and I had one social event last weekend that I went to and I was afraid-afraid to, uh, t-t- to introduce myself to anybody there. So I did some, but not-not very much.

Alerted to Walt's implicit self-blame for not following through on their plan for him to engage more fully in interactions with others, Bob begins to *externalize* "stuttering," casting it as a character with its own intentions and influence on Walt's social life. At the same time, he begins *relative influence questioning* to tease out the problem's influence on Walt:

> **Bob:** So it sounds like the stuttering has really played a role in kind of *isolating* you, even in the presence of other people. It tends to *silence* you in a way, and . . . ?
>
> **Walt:** Well yes, it-it's the worst part, I think. It is just, I feel so embarrassed and, . . . I just feel so bad, I guess *ashamed* when I am stuttering, es-especially so-, especially socially, that I, I just, I just don't want to go to many, I don't want to go anywhere.
>
> **Bob:** So it is as if stuttering has shamed you in the presence of others. What do you think stuttering is convincing other people to think about you? About who Walt is?
>
> **Walt:** I think they think I'm stupid. I think they think I-I-I don't have anything-anything to say, but it's . . . Because I am changing words and I'm not using . . . , I'm not saying it the way I would write it, I'm not saying words that are the best words to use, and I . . . um . . . I am so hesitant I'm sure I look very unsure of myself and I, I, I. There are just some words I w-w-would like to use, but I'm afffraid to t-t-t, afraid to touch them and t-to-to-t-try them so I think people think I . . . especially because I don't talk, and I- when I talk I don't make sense sometimes, and I don't use the . . . I avoid so much that just I think people think I'm very, either dumb or weird or incapable or just not-not-not-not very bright.

Drawing on Walt's description of the censoring impact of stuttering on his speech with others ("I'm not saying the words that are the best to use"), Bob extends the metaphoric depiction of the problem to capture this additional influence:

> **Bob:** So it's almost as if stuttering is a severe kind of *editor* who is reaching in there and just, I can almost see it, just *redlining out* words that you would want to use. And it leaves you in kind of mute silence or having to choose another word that doesn't quite do the job that you want it to?

Walt: Yeah. Yeah. I am not spontaneous. I won't let myself be spontaneous and I. . . . It's just too scary. Um. Yeah, I don't know, I guess that's almost *worse* then the actual stuttering, and, well when I . . . Even when I don't stutter, often when I do but even when I don't stutter, people just give me this *look*. There is this very definite look of . . . they're- they are nervous, or scared, they're not, not—uh, ug—they are not sure what I am trying to say and they are just kinda k–kwi-kwi . . . they're kinda unsure of what I am saying.

Bob: So it's as if stuttering has not only had a direct effect on you, a *real effect* in the way you think about yourself, in terms of the feeling of being stupid and not being able to find the words; it's had an effect on your language, and it has had an effect on the way other people receive you, and their kind of nervousness or uneasiness or unsureness around you. And the net effect of this is a kind of, almost a *solitary confinement*, in a way, in your life.

Walt: Yeah, I think that is a good way to say it! I . . . Certainly what I feel, I am so limited, I guess I am choosing to be limited and com-c-c-c-com-ug . . . compromised.

Here Walt clearly resonates to the image of stuttering putting him in solitary confinement, but starts to tilt back subtly toward self-blame for "choosing" to be limited. Sensing that this could be a slippery slope, Bob offers a partial "as if" reframe in keeping with the discussion of stuttering's influence on Walt:

Bob: At this point it is almost as if *stuttering* is doing the choosing *for you* in terms of what settings you can be in or can't be in, or whether you can enter them spontaneously or in a kind of much more measured and guarded way. Like it's. . . .

Walt: Yeah, I mean, I *hate* it! I think that is why I hate it so much. Because I'm not . . . *I don't even know who I am* because I won't let myself try or experiment or go.

As they conclude this segment of the interview, Walt not only works with the image of stuttering as something that influences his behavior, but also strongly objects to it as something that has hijacked his capacity to choose, or even know who he really is as a person. As discussed in Chapters 8 and 10, this represents an *iMoment* in which Walt clearly begins to *protest* against the influence of stuttering, and in this sense contest its role as the dominant narrative of his life. The stage is therefore set for his more active resistance against stuttering's isolating and silencing role in his life, as expressed in some additional sessions of counseling focused on *experimenting with experience* by speaking out in settings that had previously intimidated him.

Audible Progress

Bob: Hi Walt, it's good to see you again this week. We've had a couple of sessions now since, um, I remember your first vivid descriptions of the way in which stuttering seemed to be dictating your life. And you've been pushing back against that almost dictatorial control, and I'm, I'm just very interested in how that, that resistance is going for you this week *(inviting an expansion of the story of resistance)*.

Walt: Well it's still very scary. It's not what I'm used to doing. But I have days when I'm willing to take more risks, and um, and um, have had s-some success. I don't know that I am really s-s-stuttering any less but I am p-p-p-participating more . . . uh, a little.

Bob: Uh-*huh*! Tell me about some of those times when you've taken that risk of participation, right. Even if the stuttering makes an appearance, you're somehow also making more of an appearance on the social stage?

Walt: Well, the best example that I was actually k . . . I stuttered, but I was kinda proud of the fact that I answered a question in class, the other day in a class that I normally don't say anything. I think the inst… the teacher was really surprised actually, kinda taken back that I even raised my hand. Umm . . . .

Bob: So, you weren't even called on necessarily but you kind of volunteered yourself to answer a question.

Walt: Yeah, it was like *jumping off a cliff*. I just, I didn't know what would happen. I stuttered, but I didn't stutter as much as I thought I would . . . which was really a surprise. It was kind of *nice*, but it was kind of *scary*.

As Bob prompts for a specific example of a "unique outcome," a time Walt took the risk of "making an appearance on the social stage," Walt immediately recalls boldly volunteering to answer a question in an executive class he is taking. Not only does he sketch out the *action iMoment* arising from this experiment, but he also consolidates it with a *reflective iMoment*, recognizing the "nice but scary" feeling that accompanied it, like adventurously "jumping off a cliff." Eager to validate and extend this reflection, Bob recalls vaguely that Walt was a competitive swimmer in college, and so nudges the metaphor in this direction:

Bob: It felt kind of good and exhilarating, like *taking a dive from a high board* at a swimming pool, or kind of . . .

Walt: Yeah, it *did*! I felt like an out of body experience, like *it didn't feel like me at all*. But I, um. But it was, I guess, exhilarating, but it was *still so different* that it, is what I mean, it was an *out* of body kind of thing.

Bob: Sort of hard to wrap your mind around it. "Is it really me doing this? Is it the familiar Walter I know and love, or is it a different person making an appearance here?", almost.

Walt: Yeah, it was *fun*, but it was just, it was very . . . it was *weird*. It was so *new*, I guess.

Bob: Hard to know what to make of it?

Walt: Yeah.

The Challenge of Change

As is often the case when change begins to happen, it can be hard to construe, hard to make sense of. Walt recognizes this, and underscores the "weird, new" feeling of behaving so differently, almost an "out of body" feeling. Just as in the research discussed in

Chapter 7, he seems to feel the *cognitive anxiety* that comes with stepping beyond his personal constructs of who he has long been, even though it also feels exhilarating to do so. Bob therefore holds the focus on this reflective i-Moment to help Walt step toward a *reconceptualization* of how he achieved this great leap forward:

> **Bob:** How did you build yourself up to the point of taking that running jump into this kind of unknown element?
>
> **Walt:** I think a lot of it is based on what we talked about, of realizing how *sick* I am of doing it the old way. I just, I almost don't care what people think, and I-I guess I wanted to u-use, like we've talked about, I wanted to use that audience to . . . I wanted to use them instead of being scared by, I just wanted to practice to see what happened.
>
> **Bob:** Ahhhh, for you to use the audience rather than for you to be used by stuttering in a way. To be able to really say, "Here's a group of people who I can use to make an appearance in a different way than stuttering has let me do in the past."
>
> **Walt:** There was another part that was really strange too. I almost . . . I felt good about it and I was more fluent then I thought I would be, but um. . . . This is really *strange*. I really, I don't even want to talk about it, I guess but I . . . I almost felt guilty for being . . . I don't know, I just felt *guilty*. I mean it's, I know it sounds strange, uneasy, I know that's not the word, but *it didn't feel like me*. It was fun, but it didn't feel like me.

The Paradox of Progress

As often happens, Walt describes the change he is beginning to perform with a curious sense of ambivalence. On the one hand, he experiences the "fun" of taking a wild leap into more fluid public speaking, but on the other hand, he feels a kind of "uneasiness" or "guilt" about doing so. In constructivist terms, this is entirely understandable: in stepping toward fluency, he has also stepped away from a familiar construction of himself, seemingly contradicting an old and apparently "authentic" identity of himself as a person who stutters. This is what personal construct theorists term *guilt* (Kelly, 1955/1991), and what many disfluent participants in our study of speaking roles described when they tried to imagine themselves as more fluent speakers (see DiLollo, Manning, & Neimeyer, 2003 and 2005 summarized in Chapter 7). To help Walt consolidate this shift more fully, Bob therefore holds a kind of "magnifying glass" over the *constructive revision* part of this experience cycle, extending the reflective iMoment to capture more of what Walt was feeling, sensing, and doing in this moment of change.

> **Bob:** It doesn't fit with the image of *who I was* and in some way am supposed to be, right? I am supposed to be this person who stutters and . . . ?
>
> **Walt:** Yeah, I guess maybe that's *it*, yeah. I'm not sure, I guess that was . . . would be it, maybe.
>
> **Bob:** And you say, as you did this you stuttered a little bit, but less than you might have expected?
>
> **Walt:** Yeah, I mean I had a really long time, hard block where nothing happened but I was able to have enough presence of mind. . . . I didn't really use the techniques very well but I was able to grab g-grab on to them a little bit.
>
> **Bob:** Tell me about that. What kind of techniques or skills that we have worked on did you make use of in that setting to push away from the hold that stuttering had on you, and to really take a leap into something new, exhilarating?
>
> **Walt:** Well I just . . . changed the nature of the stuttering w-w-w . . . where I went like that, where I changed the nature of it, where *I gave myself permission* to stutter easier. Which I can do in easier situations, but I've never done in that situation before, that's a hard. . . .
>
> **Bob:** Yeah, yeah, that's really something! That's really a *sparkling moment*, to be able to say, to put these skills to use, not in a therapy setting but in a real life setting. And to say, "Yeah, I can push back against stuttering, I can modify it, I can change it, and not just have it change me."

Frequently when progress first occurs in a communication disorder, clients minimize the importance of what has taken place. Thus, even though Walt had evocatively described the new and exhilarating feeling of speaking out, in a sense "talking back" to stuttering's influence on his life, he finds himself mitigating the significance of this action iMoment, as if to protect himself from disappointment. Bob therefore seeks to enlarge the moment by anchoring it in the perceptions of significant witnesses to the new narrative that Walt is beginning to perform:

> **Walt:** It was just a *tiny thing* though, I don't, I don't think it was a. . . .You know, it was good, but it is so rare that I can do that. I don't know how much to make of it, you know?

> **Bob:** Well let's make as much of it as we can, shall we? Let's *celebrate* this! The image I get is like beginning to put just a little bit of daylight between you and stuttering. Just a few degrees of separation in a way that starts to let you sense yourself in a different way.

> **Walt:** Yeah, it's just a tiny thing. I want to, I tend to want to discount it because it was so small. But it was, as you described, it was *different.*

> **Bob:** Was it big enough that others noticed it as well?

> **Walt:** I don't know that they understood. I think I would have to explain it to them. You know my, my *wife* would understand that because she has been here, and *you* understand it, but I don't think most of my teachers or most of my classmates would understand what happened there.

> **Bob:** The kind of thing that your wife or me or someone would understand about it—who are really on the inside with you—is that we could see this, this, almost a sense of *guilt* of stepping out of the old roles. Others wouldn't see that, but what they would see and they would hear was maybe Walt raising his hand or Walt answering a question for the first time.

> **Walt:** Yeah, right. Also, I made a couple phone calls this week that I wouldn't have ever made before.

Bob: Huh! (*sounding surprised*)

Walt: And on a couple of them I didn't stutter *at all*, and I normally would have thought, I would have predicted I would have, but I didn't. Others, you know, that were harder, I stuttered quite a bit but I, but I made the phone calls, which is something I wouldn't have ever done six weeks ago.

Shift Happens

As Walt begins to spontaneously recall further innovative moments in which he acted outside the frame of his dominant narrative of stuttering, Bob underscores these, then shifts to the reflective level, prompting Walt to consider their broader significance for his sense of self:

Bob: So speaking in class, making a couple of phone calls, where previously you would have just forgone the calls, not even made them. . . .

Walt: Yeah, my wife would have made them. I would have asked her to.

Bob: Yeah, yeah, yeah, yeah. So you're really beginning to have more of a *voice* in your life, on the telephone, in public settings.

Walt: A little bit, yeah.

Bob: What do these things suggest about *who you are*? What kind of *strengths* you're drawing on to accomplish this?

Walt: Well I guess . . . that I am tougher than I thought I was. I always knew I had things to say, but I think, this sounds strange too, I go back to the fact when I was in college when I was on the *swimming team*. And it really made me feel so good, I had great success, *unexpected success*, because I worked really hard and I was in the pool first and out of the pool last and was *very, very determined* and persistent, and it, it, it . . . it turned out that I broke a lot of uh-uh-uh-uh, of *records* that I didn't know I could break, I didn't know I had that ability. That experience was really helpful, and applies to this situation, I think.

Bob: I'm *really* getting the sense of that, and I even have some tingles up my spine as I hear that, and the way you describe, for example, answering the question in class, the kind of *leaping off* into something new. . . . I almost get the sense of the diver who is poised there on the edge of the pool and then suddenly jumps in and takes off and . . .

Walt: Yeah! I almost just wanted to *go for it* and see what happened, to kind of perform an *experiment*.

Bob: To break your own record, I guess!

Linking spontaneously to the proud era of Walt's college swim team victories, client and clinician bring to bear these dependable strengths on his persistent efforts to dive into speaking situations in a new way, and push his performance beyond what he once thought possible.

Re-Writing the Story

The growing edge of change is seldom even, of course, and two steps forward can be followed by one step back. But as Walt continued—ever more boldly—to step toward rather than away from previously anxiously avoided situations, using familiar speech modification tools in a more comfortable, natural way, the evolution in his sense of self and social behavior was unmistakable. The following dialogue represents the sort of *reconceptualization iMoment* (Gonçalves, Matos, & Santos, 2010) in which a client is able to not only *perform change* but also *narrate* it, in the sense of being able to recognize the shift from the past, problem-saturated story to a current one marked by much more personal agency over the problem, and to relate just how this change occurred.

Bob: Well it's good to talk with you once more, and it sounds to me as if we are headed into our last couple of conversations, after the strides you have been making in really reclaiming your life from the grip of stuttering. And I am just wondering if you can give me a bit of an update on how that's going for you?

Walt: Uh . . . I . . . I've had more fluent, I mean I've always been more fluent in our therapy sessions, but I'm finding I'm more fluent, not every day, it's still variable (*gesturing in a "roller coaster" way*), but, uh, I'm more fluent more often. And I think I'm getting a little bit *used* to it, and I think others are kind of expecting it more often, and that's good. But it also, I feel sometimes pressure to maintain that fluency; not trip up and fail or however you think of it like that. But generally, I feel more *confident*, more *powerful*, more *a part of my surroundings*.

Bob: Uh huh. Really more *connected* to things instead of that sort of isolation that you described early on, where you would silence yourself at the party or not even go. Now you're making more of an appearance in your life, it seems.

Walt: Yes. Yeah, I don't—actually, on a couple of occasions I've expressed myself. . . . I don't know that I've been *obnoxious*, but I mean I've enjoyed my fluency so much *I don't always know when to shut up now!* Because I, maybe I'm just overdoing it a bit, cause I feel this *power* that I've never experienced much of before.

Bob: A real power that you've never experienced. And I'm really enjoying that image of you just being so powerful that you're almost a little bit obnoxious!

Walt: Yeah, and I've not said things for so long now that I have, I feel like I have a lot to say!

The Archeology of an Alternative History

As this bright new image of Walt as a comfortable and assertive speaker begins to emerge into full view, Bob seeks to build a foundation for it by excavating a previously buried history capable of supporting this structure. This entails the recruitment of witnesses from Walt's past who would have known that he had what it took to wrestle his life and relationships back from the hold of stuttering, and claim it more fully as his own.

> **Bob:** Uh huh. A *lot* to say. Who in your life do you think would have most appreciated that you could get to a point that you had this to say, and were quite able to say it in the powerful way that you are? Who would have seen that coming, or know that you had it in you to do that?
>
> **Walt:** I think my *mother* would have. I think she . . . I don't know, I just, maybe I think mothers think that way, but I just felt she knew that I was stronger than I was showing.
>
> **Bob:** What could she have told me about Walter if I had said, "Tell me a little bit about your son. What is it that is going to give him the strength to persevere even against the obstacles that life throws in his way? What could you tell me about him?"
>
> **Walt:** I think she would have just said, "He's not stupid."
>
> **Bob:** He's not stupid.
>
> **Walt:** That "I know that he is, um, maybe more talent-talented than he knows; and has things to contribute that he's not yet doing, not yet contributing." I think my *swimming coach* would have seen the toughness and the strength, the determination to not give in. I think he would have known that.
>
> **Bob:** That kind of perseverance to really break the records, to not simply to take a few laps in the pool, but really to push yourself.
>
> **Walt:** Yeah, just stick with it. Um, I think my *close friends* who knew me, I mean that's maybe why they were my friends. I think they knew I was, not only wasn't stupid, but that I was . . . maybe not just dependable for them but *dependable for myself*. I mean I, that *I wouldn't quit on me* either. Although it certainly seemed that I had every reason to at one time.
>
> **Bob:** Yeah. Yeah. Stuttering seemed to *give* you that reason and yet you've really kind of said *no* to that, and you know,

you're saying in a way, "I can depend on myself, and others can depend on me, and me on them, in a different way than before."

Walt: Yeah. I think that . . . It's still *new* to me, and it, I'm still unsure and I think other people aren't necessarily used to this, who I am, or who I'm becoming, and it's . . . it takes some adjustment on their part, um, because it's very different.

Back to the Future

With this alternative past in fuller view, clearly validated by the constructions of Walt's mother, coach and friends, Bob then attempts to prompt for the alternative future narrative it makes possible. In a sense, this initiates a new experience cycle by cuing up new *anticipations* of possible preferred outcomes in light of his reconstructed sense of self.

Bob: Yeah. Let's see if we can extend that a little bit. Let's see if we can look in the dusty crystal ball of the future a little bit. Beyond today, beyond this period of initial successes, in kind of reclaiming your life from stuttering, just imagine what your life may look like if you continue to move down this road in the direction of greater power, greater dependability. Right? What kind of image comes to you of this life that you might yet lead?

Walt: Well, with my career I've always wanted to give workshops and presentations and I've refused to do that. To put myself in front of a group, and I . . . I don't know, it sounds crazy almost. But I think that . . . I think that as I become w-what I maybe can be, what I think I can be, I think that I might enjoy doing that. Not just be able to do that well, maybe better than I thought I could, better than I've seen other people do it, but I think I have a *passion*, and uh . . . Maybe I have things to say that I can not only say well, but say it . . . d-d-do a good job communicating.

Bob: Persuasively, powerfully, passionately, right? To really *literally* have a place on stage?

Walt: Yeah. That sounds so *strange* to me to even say that but I think maybe that that's a possibility in the future.

Bob: And that's a very different future than the future that stuttering had planned for you.

Walt: Oh yeah. I mean I will, I wouldn't have been there. I wouldn't have allowed myself.

Bob: *Hugely* different. Is there anybody else in your life now that needs to learn about these interesting new developments and possibilities in your life?

Walt: Huh. Yeah, well . . . I think that my colleagues, and, um . . . I'd like to tell them about it, and *show* them. I'd like to go back to some of the previous speech clinicians I've had and tell them that even though I didn't do what maybe they wanted me to do, that in the long run that's how it came out. I'd like to . . . to let them know who I am now.

Bob: Using some of the techniques and skills that they taught you but also really pushing yourself in ways that they couldn't have envisioned.

Walt: Yeah, so they could see the full process of that . . . change that took twenty years, that took a long time. That it is possible.

Bob: Well, I have certainly enjoyed seeing the part of the process that I have been privileged to witness, and take part in as a very interested spectator. And I really want to join that audience for the performance of this new Walt that we see emerging on stage here, and just, uh, express my *appreciation* to you and my *respect* for you for the way in which you are changing this, this whole narrative of your life. And it feels good to be a reader of that new narrative.

Walt: Thanks for your help!

Coda: Re-Writing the Self-Narrative

As Walt's case suggests, separating the person from the problem—whether it is a hearing problem, an articulation difficulty, disfluency, or other communication disorder—through externalization can promote a clearer recognition of the relative influence that each has, or could have on the other, in a way that resists stigmatizing and pathologizing discourses that view the client as broken or deficient. Instead, the narrative tropes described in the previous chapter and illustrated in this one assume a respectful view of clients as resourceful, resilient, and ultimately resistant to the reductive impact of the problem in their lives.

From this perspective, clinician and client actively foster experimenting with experience, attending to innovative moments of protest, action, and reflection that ultimately scaffold a reconceptualization of a more competent and hopeful self. (See Figure 11–1, a conceptual map of Walt's therapy.) In the course of such adaptive counseling, which builds upon the technical devices and skills that are an equally important part of treatment, clients can succeed in winning back their lives from the dominant narrative of their deficiency, and live into a future that is not determined by their past.

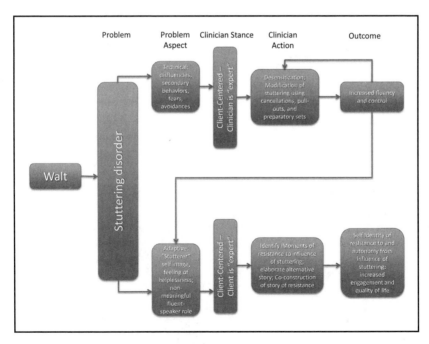

Figure 11–1. A conceptual map of Walt's therapy.

References

DiLollo, A., Manning, W. H., & Neimeyer, R. A. (2003). Cognitive anxiety as a function of speaker role for fluent speakers and persons who stutter. *Journal of Fluency Disorders, 28*(3), 167–186. doi:10.1016/S0094-730X(03)00043-3

DiLollo, A., Manning, W. H., & Neimeyer, R. A. (2005). Cognitive complexity as a function of speaker role for adult persons who stutter. *Journal of Constructivist Psychology, 18*(3), 215–236. doi:10.1080/10720530590948773

Gonçalves, M. M., Matos, M., & Santos, A. (2010). Narrative therapy and the nature of "innovative moments" in the construction of change. In J. D. Raskin, S. K. Bridges, & R. A. Neimeyer (Eds.), *Studies in meaning* (Vol. 4). New York, NY: Pace University Press.

Kelly, G. A. (1955/1991). *The psychology of personal constructs.* New York, NY: Routledge.

Neimeyer, R. A. (2000). Narrative disruptions in the construction of self. In R. A. Neimeyer & J. D. Raskin (Eds.), *Constructions of disorder: Meaning making frameworks for psychotherapy* (pp. 207–241). Washington, DC: American Psychological Association.

12

ADAPTIVE COUNSELING AND INNOVATIVE MOMENTS: A CASE ILLUSTRATION

By now the concepts of *adaptive counseling* (see Chapter 3) and *innovative moments* or iMoments (see Chapters 8 & 10) should be familiar. The former refers to interventions that address murkier problems often implicating changes in the *problem-solver*, rather than the relative clarity of technical interventions targeting concrete aspects of the *problem behavior* or communication disorder only. And the latter concept refers to those "sparkling moments" of possibility when the client begins to resist the domination of the problem story of disability, and (re)claim a measure of self-respect or hope that previously seemed inaccessible.

But how do these concepts apply in an actual case of therapy for a significant communication disorder, across a series of treatment sessions that include technical as well as adaptive goals? In this chapter we'll seek to illustrate the practical value of thinking in these terms when faced with a complex case that had "stalled"—or even seemed destined for failure—when approached at a merely technical level. Drawing on a narrative conceptualization of the client's challenges as well as a strengths-based assessment of his competencies and interests, the clinicians ultimately sought to ally with the person behind the problem, to reach beyond its constraints to a life of fuller engagement with the person he had previously been. The story unfolded in a university clinic, and began with a consultation following a serious cerebrovascular accident (CVA) suffered by a popular professor on that same campus.

The Case of the Aphasic Professor

George is a 62-year-old white male. He lives with his wife, Amy, in a small college town. They have a 27-year-old son who is married and lives in California. George had been a biology professor for over 30 years prior to his left-hemisphere stroke approximately two years prior to the date of this case study. Following the stroke, George has had severe weakness and moderate paralysis on his right side (he had no use of his right hand and he needed a cane to walk), significant dysarthria, and a severe expressive aphasia. His communication was characterized by poor word-finding skills, poor intelligibility, and an absence of initiating any verbal communication.

George had been receiving speech-language therapy at the university clinic in his hometown for the past two years. Given his lack of progress and length of time post-stroke, it is unlikely that George would have continued to receive services for this length of time if it had not been at the university clinic where he was known from his days as a professor. When I first met George, it was the start of a new semester and I was scheduled to supervise two female SLP students to work with him. As is customary in most university clinics, we inherited George's treatment plan from the supervisor and students who had worked with him the previous semester. The treatment report was not encouraging, indicating that George had made little progress, appeared depressed and angry, and was frequently noncompliant, both during sessions and with any homework assignments. George's treatment plan included drills for improving his intelligibility (repetition of simple words), cueing for eliciting naming, using flash cards in a naming task, naming common objects, and simple, scripted conversations about pictures.

Watching the first session with George was painful! He was as non-compliant, depressed, and angry as the report had indicated. The students were unsure of how to handle him, so they reverted to their most familiar clinical script—stick to the lesson plan at all costs and provide positive encouragement using their best, over-the-top *"Good job!"* (with a lot of nervous giggles). I decided then that we needed to do something very different because this was definitely not working!

From Technical Therapy to Adaptive Counseling

When the students and I met to discuss their next session with George, I suggested to them that we needed to re-conceptualize George and his treatment plan—we needed to think about things differently. His current plan had been designed based on George's disorder and what the "expert" speech-language pathologist knew were evidence-based treatments for those deficits. This plan was designed to address the *technical* aspects of George's problem but did not consider the *adaptive* aspects. The problem was that George was being affected as much by the adaptive aspects of his problem as he was by the technical. We needed to start thinking of George in a holistic manner, putting the *person* and his *story* at the center of the plan—which then made George (and his wife) the "experts."

We started down this new track by spending some time talking with Amy, George's wife. She typically could not be at therapy sessions because of her work schedule, but she made time to meet with us. We asked Amy about their life, about what George does, how they communicate, the other significant people in George's life, and what problems they were encountering since the stroke. We also asked about what George was like before the stroke, the things he liked to do, what his communication was like, and what things he didn't like.

What we found out was that George was an intelligent, patient man, who liked to work on his computer, read journals, browse the Web, and watch "scientific" shows on TV. He also had a good sense of humor, enjoyed playing card games, and used to keep in touch with his son in California via e-mail. We also learned that one thing that irritated George was "giggling sorority girls"—a product of teaching undergraduate biology classes! In contrast, after the stroke, George was depressed and did nothing all day but watch TV, without even appearing to care what was on. Amy did tell us that she came home one day to find that George had tried to use his computer but that he had been unsuccessful because he couldn't use the mouse due to the weakness in his right hand and arm. She said that he refused to even go near the computer after that.

A Spark of Innovation

As we built an understanding of George's story—as a husband, father, scholar—we began to understand why George was acting the way he was and the role that we, his clinicians, we playing in it. Essentially, therapy served as a constant reminder to George of what he couldn't do, as well as placing him in the care of young college girls who often responded to him as they would to a child—and giggled—possibly his worst nightmare! We also, however, found an *action iMoment*—when George tried the computer. Although he didn't succeed, this indicated that he wanted to do something other than sit around all day; that he wanted to get back to doing something that he'd enjoyed prior to the stroke. Triggered by this iMoment, we studied George's stories from before the stroke and after the stroke to see if we could build on this attempt by George to break away from the story of helplessness and depression that the stroke had written for him. What we realized was that much of what George liked to do prior to the stroke—using the computer, playing card games, watching specific TV shows—might still be available to him but had gotten lost in the trauma and depression of his physical changes.

In Search of a New Deal

To elaborate this alternative story, we redesigned George's treatment plan to explore some of the activities that he enjoyed prior to his stroke. We decided to start by playing poker, a relatively easy card game that Amy told us George had played before. When we introduced the poker game into George's session, we asked him to help review the rules of the game with the clinicians, giving him the excuse that the girls were not sure of the rules. The clinicians would say things like, "So, a full house is when you have a pair and three of a kind, is that right?" and they would wait for his response. A number of times they would "get it wrong" so that George needed to correct them, usually by saying "No" and pointing to a list of possible poker hands. In this way, the clinicians were able to actively position George as the "expert" and in control, while also building a cooperative relationship (and the clinicians no longer responded to George as a child). The poker games formed the core of the sessions, but various goals were incorporated into the games. For example, we used plastic chips to "bet" on the games, so George had to practice counting out loud and communicating his "bet." In addition, simple conversations were engaged in during the game, which were often pre-planned by the clinicians but some also occurred spontaneously (although George still did not initiate). We encouraged Amy to play cards with George at home and she reported that they started doing this frequently at night instead of watching TV, restoring a valued form of relating that had become a collateral casualty of the stroke.

Changing the Channel

In order to help George have some choices for activities at home, we started working with him on playing solitaire with the playing cards. Again, this was a game that was familiar to him and he was able to pick it up quickly. We also worked on helping George read the TV guide so that he might select programs that were of interest to him. We showed the TV guide to George and asked him what was difficult about reading it. We knew that he could read many single words and sentences from his previous "technical" therapy. Through pointing, gestures, and saying "Too much," George was able to tell us that the small, crowded pages of the TV guide were confusing for him. By working through the guide with George, we created a simplified, enlarged version with his favorite channels on it. We worked with George to ensure that he could read it accurately and that he could also read his watch accurately so that he could plan out when he was going to watch TV. Throughout this process, the clinicians would ask questions about the TV shows that George liked, cueing him as needed to facilitate his word finding.

Rewriting the Story of Disability

An interesting transformation began to take place as we instituted these new treatment procedures with George: (1) Amy reported less depressive symptoms at home, (2) George became much more engaged in therapy sessions and completed all homework tasks, often going beyond the assigned task, and (3) he began to display signs of the sense of humor that Amy had described as part of his story prior to the stroke, frequently teasing the clinicians about their taste in TV programs or how poorly they played poker. George appeared to be reclaiming parts of his old story and merging them into a new story of resisting the limiting effects of the stroke. At our meeting at the end of the semester, we re-told this alternative story to George and Amy, and invited Amy to provide her re-telling of the story as well.

The following semester, George returned and the same clinicians were assigned to him again (by design, as we considered their relationship with George to be a significant factor in his progress). Amy reported that George had continued to reconstruct his story over the break, enjoying a visit from their son, whom George had not seen since immediately after his stroke two years before. She said that they had all gone out to eat one night, something that George had previously refused to do.

We decided that, as George was now proficient at playing both poker and solitaire, we needed to try something new. So we asked George if he would be willing to try using the computer. At first he just said, "Can't" and shook his head. We asked him if he would be willing to just try an experiment with it. Although skeptical, the strong therapeutic alliance that the clinicians had built with him over the past few months meant that he trusted them, so he agreed. We started by getting him to just play solitaire on the computer. This had several advantages, as it was a familiar activity (he had been playing the same game with the cards for a while now) as well as being a relatively simple motor task as he built competence using his left hand to control the mouse. Being careful not to lapse back into the relatively meaningless, *"Good job"* responses, the clinicians quietly encouraged George and supported his efforts. We also had Amy make sure that their computer at home was set up so that George could easily access it and use the mouse with his left hand.

It did not take long for George to master using the mouse with his left hand. Within two weeks of starting to use the computer to play solitaire, George was browsing the web, at first with guidance from the clinicians, then alone at home. Throughout these activities, the clinicians engaged George in short conversations, often asking questions about web pages he chose to visit or asking him to find out specific information by doing a web search. Although he continued to have word-finding difficulties and a moderate level of dysarthria, George's *communication* had improved significantly, even including an occasional initiation of verbal interactions, both with the clinicians and at home with Amy.

Composing Life Out of Loss

As his computer skills improved, we asked George if he would like to try using email. He readily agreed and immediately wanted to e-mail his son. The clinicians helped George compose a series of e-mails to his son, and it became the first thing that we did in each session—check to see if he had an email from his son, read it, and compose and send a reply. Although composing and typing e-mails was difficult for George, he liked doing it as it represented a further reclaiming of his story from the effects of the stroke. Each session, the clinicians assigned George homework to compose parts of an e-mail to send to his son. On one occasion, when he showed the clinicians a longer than usual e-mail that he had constructed, they asked "How were you able to do this all by yourself?" With a gleam in his eye and his crooked smile, he said, "Work hard!"

Before we ended therapy with George, approximately one year after implementing his new plan, he engaged in a rather remarkable endeavor that, even just a few weeks earlier, would have seemed unlikely. One day in therapy, he indicated to the clinicians that he wanted to do a specific search on the computer. He sat down and went directly to a web site about cruises and he said, "Going . . . this" and pointed to the cruise ship. Impressed, the clinicians asked, "You want to go on a cruise?" "No," he replied, "Going!" He then pulled out a piece of paper that was a printout of a series of e-mails between George and his son. Some of George's e-mails didn't make sense, but his son had patiently asked for clarification and, clearly, George eventually got his message across. On George's suggestion, he and his son had planned to surprise Amy with a cruise for their wedding anniversary that was a few months away. Despite his struggles to get it done, this small taste of independence and initiative again fed into George's reclamation and reconstruction of his personal narrative.

Throughout George's therapy, Amy had been highly engaged, despite not being able to be at many sessions due to her work schedule. Towards the end of the semester, however, as we were planning on terminating George's therapy, we asked Amy if she could join us for his last two sessions. Our intention here was to "sell" George's re-constructed story and engage in a series of tellings and retellings to help place the story on a solid foundation. We talked about what George could do, what he liked and disliked, and what he had given to us by trusting and working with us. Amy told of reclaiming a relationship that she thought was lost—everyone cried! Before they left, Amy took us aside and hugged each of us and said, "You gave me my husband back. Thank you!"

Interestingly, in many ways, George's technical gains were relatively limited as he continued to struggle with naming objects, word finding, and dysarthria, and I suspect that he would have performed only mildly better on the technical tasks that were part of his therapy prior to the changes that we implemented. Despite this, his adaptive gains were striking and changed his life, as he reached beyond the dark hold of sullen anger and depression to reclaim a sparkling sense of self and loving connection that had once seemed lost to his disorder.

Conceptual Map of George's Therapy

Having read George's story, let's take a closer look at how his therapy mapped onto the conceptual map introduced in Chapter 8 (Figure 12–1). Following the "technical" branch, we note the specific speech and language deficits that George was left with following his stroke. Given that he was two years post-stroke, it seemed unlikely that George was going to make any new gains in these areas of deficit, yet those were the only aspects that his original treatment plan focused on—unwittingly condemning George to being stuck in the loop between "clinician action" and "outcome." This is an all-too-frequent occurrence in speech-language pathology, where clinicians become so focused on the technical aspects of the problem that they forget that clients are real people, trying to function in the real world.

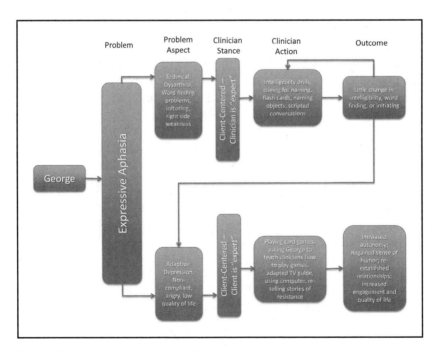

Figure 12–1. A conceptual map of George's therapy.

If we turn to the adaptive branch of the map, we can see the consequences of focusing exclusively on the technical issues that George faced. Not only did George have to deal with the adaptive consequences of his stroke—his loss of function, loss of career, loss of independence, and real challenges to his relationships—but he also had to deal with the feedback from the technical "solutions" to his speech and language deficits—his continued failure at even simple speech and language tasks and being treated, in many ways, like a child. The result was anger, depression, and isolation, and an inability to tap into any remaining strengths that he might have possessed. Changing George's therapy to focus on adaptive rather than technical issues enabled him to free himself from the impact of his technical limitations and find those residual strengths and re-author a preferred identity that returned him, at least in part, to the man that he had once been.

The case described here didn't involve any "counseling" in the way that many clinicians think of it—sitting down face-to-face with someone and talking about his or her problems. We didn't "do counseling" with anyone in this case—even though I suspect that Amy might have benefited from it had the opportunity arisen. It is hard to deny, however, that by approaching our work with George through a constructivist counseling framework, we were able to have a profound, positive impact on his life and the lives of his family. So, maybe we did "do counseling" after all!

13

THE CREDULOUS APPROACH AND RECONSTRUCTION: A CASE ILLUSTRATION

The Perfect Child

Bella, a 3-month-old girl, was tested with electrophysiologic measures. Otoacoustic emissions were absent, tympanograms normal, and acoustic reflexes were present, although elevated. The electrophysiologic thresholds were consistent with moderate to severe bilateral hearing loss.

When informed of the results, Mr. Howell, Bella's father responded angrily, saying, *"I don't know why I agreed to this. I know how you guys work. Now I guess you are going to tell us that she needs some expensive treatment or hearing aids or something! I know she can hear me, everyone tells me I have to be quiet or I'll wake the baby, and, dammit, they're right! The least bit of noise and she wakes up!"*

In Defense of Core Constructs

How do you interpret Mr. Howell's reaction, and how might you react to this response? In most cases, this reaction would be termed "denial" with the suggestion that Mr. Howell needs to "accept" his daughter's hearing loss and "move on." Suggesting this to him, however, might be problematic and simply feed his anger. If we look at Mr. Howell's reaction in terms of our constructivist counseling framework, however, we might be able to see a different way of understanding it and, therefore, of helping.

We can start by thinking in terms of technical and adaptive aspects of the problem. Certainly, there are technical aspects that need to be taken care of that relate specifically to the child's hearing. Implementing these, however, may be quite difficult until the adaptive issues related to Mr. Howell's (and possibly Mrs. Howell's) reactions to the diagnosis have been addressed. These adaptive issues are the driving force behind the father's reaction.

In Chapter 8 we suggested that the encompassing "therapeutic stance" of the constructivist counseling framework is to "place the client in the role of the expert" and take a *"credulous approach"* (Raskin & Morano, 2004) of openness and acceptance in order to understand how the client is presently experiencing the world. In this case, we need to allow Mr. and Mrs. Howell to be the "experts" regarding their everyday experiences of Bella's hearing behavior and we need to be open and accepting of their experiences, despite the results of our more formal testing. How this might inform your response to Mr. Howell might look something like this: *"Well, Mr. Howell, I can tell that you are very frustrated, and I can understand that; particularly if you are seeing things that tell you that Bella is hearing better than our tests indicate. I'm really interested in what you are observing that tell you that her hearing is okay. You certainly know her a lot better than we do!"* Then follow with, *"Could you tell me about these experiences?"* Here you are looking for a "thick description" of Mr. Howell's experiences, acting as a curious listener, asking open-ended questions, and prompting Mr. Howell to provide more information.

Central to the constructivist counseling framework is the concept of the "personal narrative." Trying to understand Mr. Howell's response to his daughter's diagnosis from this perspective, you can ask yourself: *"What is his 'story'? What is the 'dominant narrative' that is driving this response?"* For Mr. Howell, it might be that his story about Bella is of a "perfect" child, and his projected story of Bella's and his family's future is heavily invested in the constructs that make up this story of the "perfect child." A story such as this, that is related to an individual's core role constructs, is not discarded easily, even in the face of evidence that it may not be completely valid (Kelly, 1955/1991). Consequently, just as a man about to be bankrupt from gambling can consider himself to be a successful gambler because he ignores the losses and only "remembers" the wins, Mr. Howell might be ignoring possible signs that Bella is not hearing and clinging to any sign that demonstrates that she can hear.

The Plot Thickens

By engaging Mr. Howell in thick descriptions of his experiences with Bella, the clinician might be able to identify clues to potential iMoments. For example, in telling his story, Mr. Howell might say something like, *"Well, I can give you a real clear example of Bella hearing normally. Her favorite toy is a little soft rabbit that moves and plays music . . . and whenever it starts to play its music and move around, she laughs and smiles. She loves that toy. You see? It's like when I talk to her, she always reacts. Maybe not right away, but when I get up close to her and talk, she always smiles and reacts to my voice!"* Encouraging Mr. Howell is important at this stage, recruiting him to be a part of the solution rather than the problem, so you might respond by saying, *"These are really helpful examples, Mr. Howell. Thank you. Can you tell me any more about Bella?"* Mr. Howell might give a few more examples, saying, *"Sure. There was the time that she woke when I dropped the dish. You know . . . she was in the other room then! And she always responds to Buster, my German Shepherd, when he barks. Its funny, you know, 'cause she hates Muffy, my wife's toy poodle. She can be barking all day and Bella just ignores her . . . but she loves Buster!"* As the clinician, you would note the potential for a reflection iMoment based on what Mr. Howell just described and, at an appropriate time say, *"That's really interesting . . . that Bella seems to prefer one dog over the other. Can you tell me a bit more about that?"* Mr. Howell might respond by saying, *"Well, as I said, she always responds to Buster. I guess maybe she likes his big, deep bark, compared to Muffy's little yapping! I certainly know that I do!"* As Mr. Howell pauses, if the clinician jumps in with another comment or question, it will allow him to stop there and not have to reflect further. This is a great place for the clinician to use *silence*—to force Mr. Howell to reflect and think about what he can add. After a few moments, Mr. Howell continues, *"So, yeah, she prefers Buster . . . or, at least, she responds to his barking more, I guess. I mean, she seems to like Muffy okay when she is right there playing with her. Yeah. Well. You know, I guess Buster is a lot louder than Muffy . . ."* Mr. Howell looks at the clinician, *"Do you think that is the difference?"* The clinician might respond to this question by saying, *"I guess that might be a possibility. It is probably something we should try to find out. You could really pay attention to when Bella responds to the dogs and see if you think that is what is happening. Maybe you could even experiment with some other noises—loud and soft noises— and see how Bella reacts. These wouldn't be 'clinical' tests, but I bet we could get an idea of what is happening. What do you think?"*

Listening for Exceptions

Alternatively, as you engage Mr. Howell in this conversation, recognizing his expertise in Bella's hearing behaviors and asking for more detail on potential iMoments, you might then also be able to ask a relative influence question (see Chapter 10) like, *"Thank you, Mr. Howell, for all that information. It is very helpful, and you clearly have paid a lot of attention to Bella since she was born.*

Given that, so we can make sure that we are doing everything we can for Bella, I wonder if you can think of any times at all when maybe you weren't sure if Bella was hearing well, or any examples that might have made you wonder if something wasn't right? Anything could be helpful, even if it didn't seem very significant at the time."

If Mr. Howell is able to recall any examples, asking curious questions and prompting him for more detail can help elicit the thick description that, again, may lead to reflection or even reconceptualization iMoments (Gonçalves & Ribeiro, 2012). For example, Mr. Howell might say, *"Well, there certainly isn't much . . . but if I am trying to find something that might make me question her hearing . . . I guess it could be that she doesn't seem to respond to my voice unless I am right up close to her. You know, I just wrote it off as her liking me close . . . but . . . I guess it could be that she is not hearing me as well from further away."* The clinician might respond by saying, *"Okay, thanks, Mr. Howell. I can tell that it is really hard for you to think of it like that—to think that maybe Bella might have a hearing loss. Lets keep working together to try to make sure that we are doing the best thing for Bella. I really appreciate your input so far. It has been really helpful!"*

Documenting the Shift

Following this discussion, Mr. Howell might be ready to consider the possibility that his daughter might have a hearing loss and need treatment. It is also possible, however, that this alternative story might need more time and re-telling before it becomes a viable alternative for him. In this case, scheduling to meet with Mr. and Mrs. Howell in two to three days time to allow them a couple of days to think and talk about the meeting can provide opportunities for this to take place. Before the next meeting, you could send Mr. and Mrs. Howell an e-mail that summarizes what was discussed at the last meeting, with emphasis on retelling Mr. Howell's account of Bella's hearing behaviors, both those that he suggested demonstrate her competency and those that he identified that raise

From: Anthony DiLollo
Sent: Saturday, December 07, 2013 1:18 PM
To: Howell, Michael
Subject: Bella

Dear Mr. and Mrs. Howell,

Thank you for bringing Bella to see me yesterday about her hearing. I enjoyed the opportunity to meet Bella and to explore her hearing with you. Mr. Howell, you provided many helpful examples of how well Bella seems to hear at home, such as enjoying her favorite toy that moves and plays music, and getting woken by the dropped dish. You also provided some examples that we explored together that might question Bella's ability to hear some sounds well. For example, you mentioned how Bella seems to respond better to Buster's loud barking than to Muffy's "yapping" (sorry, Mrs. Howell, but those were your husband's words!), and how she tends to respond to your voice better when you are closer.

We had discussed that maybe you could experiment with some different levels of sounds at home and see how Bella responds. I would encourage you to try this, so that when we meet again you will be able to help me work out what might be the best course of action, if any, to help Bella.

Thank you, again, for partnering with me to solve this puzzle!

Sincerely,
Anthony DiLollo

Figure 13–1. E-mail to Mr. and Mrs. Howell that served as a therapeutic document.

questions. The document might look something like the e-mail shown in Figure 13-1. (See Chapter 24 for more details on therapeutic documents.)

Note that the document does not "push" the test results or provide recommendations. The purpose of the document is to help Mr. Howell focus on the reflection iMoments and move toward a reconstruction of his story about Bella and his family, one that will encompass Bella with a hearing loss without decimating his overall narrative of her future.

Constructing Collaboration

When you meet with Mr. and Mrs. Howell again, you should start the meeting by, again, re-stating the emerging story. You might say something like, *"Thank you for coming back in and bringing Bella. She is such a beautiful little girl! So, from our last meeting, we talked about Bella's hearing and, as you know, our testing raised some concerns. But, Mr. Howell, you brought up some examples of times that you thought that Bella was hearing just fine, and those were very helpful. However, you also mentioned a number of examples of times when you noticed that there might be some question about her hearing. You mentioned . . . I am sure that you have thought a lot about this since then, so, what are your thoughts regarding Bella's hearing now?*

For the sake of our example, let's assume that Mr. and Mrs. Howell are now ready to accept that Bella may have a hearing loss. Although it is now time to begin the technical work to help Bella maximize her hearing, we cannot simply forget about her parents, nor the adaptive aspects of Bella's problem, which have now somewhat changed. Recall from Chapter 5 that, from a constructivist perspective, anxiety and fear occur when we have insufficient constructs to allow us to predict events unfolding in our environment (Kelly, 1955/1991). It is likely that Mr. and Mrs. Howell have few, if any, constructs available to them to anticipate the road ahead in dealing with Bella and her hearing loss. Consequently, providing them with information regarding Bella's hearing loss, its likely course over time (i.e., is it likely to change?), the potential treatments, and what all of this means for her speech and language, education, and overall development will be helpful. From the constructivist perspective, however, simple information is not sufficient; how the individual creates meaning from that information is the key. In this case, we are interested in helping Mr. and Mrs. Howell to take the information that we provide and reconstruct their narrative about Bella and their family in a meaningful way.

Reconstructing the Future

Practical considerations, such as providing information in small "doses" and in clear, understandable language, are important to keep in mind when providing information in situations such as this. To help Mr. and Mrs. Howell create meaningful change in their story, however, may take further work from the clinician. For example, the clinician might ask a few different relative influence questions (Epston & White, 1999) like:

- *"What will the future be like dealing with Bella's hearing loss? How is this future different from the one that you may have thought that you'd have?"*
- *"Knowing what you now know about Bella's hearing and your preferences for the future of your family, how will this knowledge affect your next step?"*
- *"Now that you know about Bella's hearing loss, who else should know about it? What difference do you think it would make to their attitude toward Bella and your family if they knew this news?"*
- *"Of the significant people in your life, who do you anticipate would have difficulty accepting the news about Bella's hearing loss?"*
- *"Of the people who knew you growing up, who would have been most likely to predict that you would be able to successfully deal with the issue of Bella's hearing loss?"*
- *"What qualities would this person have seen in you that would have led him or her to believe that you would have been able to do this?"*

As Mr. and Mrs. Howell respond to some of these questions, the clinician can build into the discussion some of the "informational counseling" that is standard practice in audiology (Clark, 1994). This information can help the Howells build constructs about the potential course of Bella's disability, the types of treatments available, and the potentially full future that she can enjoy despite her hearing loss—that she still can be that "perfect child."

Conceptual Map for the Clinical Interaction with Mr. and Mrs. Howell

Considering the conceptual map for the interaction between the audiologist and Mr. and Mrs. Howell (Figure 13–2), we see a slightly different configuration than with the maps of therapy that we looked at in Chapters 8 and 12. In this case, following the "technical" branch, we notice that there is a break between the "clinician action" and "outcome" boxes, representing the mismatch between the "expert" recommendations of the audiologist and the parents' experiences of Bella. If the audiologist continued to push her expert opinion on Mr. and Mrs. Howell, chances are that they would simply remove themselves, and Bella, from the interaction, denying or significantly delaying the help that Bella needs.

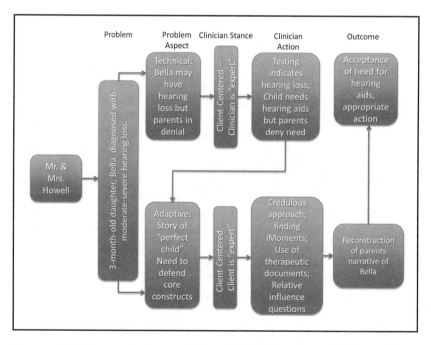

Figure 13–2. Conceptual map of the clinical interaction with Mr. and Mrs. Howell.

Following the adaptive branch, we note that Mr. and Mrs. Howell were probably already actively protecting their core constructs about Bella and her future before seeing the audiologist. This is where we ignore evidence that might invalidate our strongly held beliefs (constructs) and only attend to evidence that supports those constructs (Kelly, 1955/1991). By placing the Howells in the role of the expert and taking a credulous approach, the audiologist was able to get Mr. Howell to provide her with clues to the evidence that he had been ignoring. Then, through the audiologist's exploration of those potential iMoments with Mr. Howell, a gradual shift in his story about Bella began to occur. The clinician supported this emerging story through the use of therapeutic documents, and the Howells were eventually able to make the choice to accept the expert opinion of the audiologist ("adaptive outcome") and move toward the necessary "technical outcome."

References

Clark, J. G. (1994). Audiologists' counseling purview. In J. G. Clark & F. N. Martin (Eds.), *Effective counseling in audiology: Perspectives and practice* (pp. 1–17). Englewood Cliffs, NJ: Prentice-Hall.

Epston, D., & White, M. (1999). Termination as a right of passage: Questioning strategies for a therapy of inclusion. In R. A. Neimeyer & R. J. Mahoney (Eds.), *Constructivism in psychotherapy*. Washington, DC: American Psychological Association.

Gonçalves, M. M., & Ribeiro, A. P. (2012). Therapeutic change, innovative moments, and the reconceptualization of the self: A dialogical account. *International Journal for Dialogical Science, 6*, 81–98.

Kelly, G. A. (1955/1991). *The psychology of personal constructs*. New York, NY: Routledge.

Raskin, J. D., & Morano, L. A. (2004). Credulous approach. *Internet Encyclopedia of Personal Construct Psychology*. Retrieved September 30, 2011, from http://www.pcp-net.org/encyclopaedia/cred-appr.html

Part IV

THE CLINICIAN'S TOOLBOX

In the 12 chapters in this section of the book, we present a range of specific activities, drawn from a variety of theoretical perspectives, that clinicians can use to facilitate counseling conversations with clients who are working through any speech, language, swallowing, or hearing problem. We use the metaphor of the "toolbox" very deliberately here as that is what these activities represent: *tools.* To expand on the metaphor, we all know that tools, by themselves, are useless. They require a tradesperson who knows how to use them and what tasks each tool is suited for. Furthermore, the tradesperson must use the tools in a systematic, goal-directed way, following a plan to repair something or create something new. Our goal in these chapters is to provide readers with the knowledge of how to use these particular tools and what tasks they may be best suited for, so that they may use them within the constructivist framework described in the previous sections of the book.

14

A USER'S GUIDE TO THE CLINICIAN'S TOOLBOX

The chapters that comprise this toolbox each describe a tool that speech-language pathologists and audiologists can use to enhance externalization, spark innovative moments, and facilitate reconstruction in the course of adaptive counseling. The format of each chapter is identical to help readers build familiarity and confidence in using the toolbox. Each includes: (1) indications of *types of clients and/or situations with which the tool might be used*, as well as any contraindications for its use, (2) a list of *materials needed*, (3) a clear *description* of the tool with concrete instructions, (4) a brief *case example* that illustrates the method, how it was implemented, and what was learned from the client's responses, (5) *concluding thoughts* that consolidate the basic message of the chapter, and (6) *frequently asked questions* that address concerns or uncertainties clinicians might have about the tool and its use.

We hope that by the time readers reach this section of the book, they understand more fully why we say that the use of these tools is *not* "doing counseling." Although many clients could gain a level of insight or emotional relief simply from completing the tasks, this is not the main purpose. Instead, the tools are intended as a *starting point* for conversations between client and clinician, as a means to help clients to think about their problem in a way that is different from the default interpretations that they bring to therapy. Clinicians should not feel they need to use these tools to be "doing counseling." As we discussed in Chapter 9, *reflective listening* is the primary job of the clinician, with the goal of encouraging "thick descriptions" by the client that aid in the identification of iMoments or stories of resistance, and that remains true when using these tools. It is, in fact, the purpose for using these tools, and the creative clinician might well invent others in the course of doing so!

A particular danger for speech-language pathologists and audiologists, who are well trained and experienced in the use of standardized tests, protocols, and assessment inventories, is that the use of the tools can place them in the familiar role of "the expert," taking too active a lead in the process. Consequently, clinicians should introduce the tools tentatively, inviting clients to collaborate in shaping or modifying a particular tool to meet the needs of the moment, or to help select a tool from a subset narrowed by the clinician. In this way the clinician is able to maintain the client-centered, co-constructive nature of the counseling process.

The tools originate from a range of theoretical traditions but all fit into the constructivist, narrative therapy rationale that underlies the framework that we have been describing in this book. In this way, each of the tools in this "toolbox" can be used to facilitate various aspects of the constructivist counseling framework. For example, tools such as the *Autobiography of the Problem* (Chapter 15), *Dear John Letter* (Chapter 18), and *Chair Work* (Chapter 22) might be very useful in facilitating externalizing conversations with clients. Alternatively, tools such as *The Story Mountain* (Chapter 16), *Play Therapy* (Chapter 23), and *Therapeutic Documents* (Chapter 24) might be helpful in promoting co-construction and "selling" the client's emerging story.

The tools were selected to offer a range of potentially useful methods for nearly any client dealing with any type of problem. For example, some tools are more suited to younger clients, such as *The Story Mountain* (Chapter 16), *Drawing* (Chapter 17), and *Play Therapy* (Chapter 23), whereas others are more suited to adolescent or adult clients, such as the *Downward Arrow* (Chapter 19), *Mindfulness* (Chapter 20), and *Chair Work* (Chapter 22). Similarly, some are useful for clients who would have difficulty with complex verbal tasks (e.g., *Drawing, Play Therapy*, and *Therapeutic Documents*) while others might suit clients who enjoy creative endeavors (e.g., *Autobiography of the Problem, Drawing, Self Characterization*, and *Experimenting with Experience*). Ultimately, the point of having many methods at our disposal is to place us in the best position to select the right tool for a given job.

We hope that clinicians and students, along with their clients, will find this array of tools to be interesting, enticing, and fun to experiment with. We encourage readers to study the case examples included in each chapter, as these provide insights into how the tools might best be used for the maximum benefit of the client. Lastly, we want to remind clinicians that, despite what the hardware stores might like you to believe, it is the felicitous combination of getting the right tools in the right hands that leads to a job well done, rather than the tools themselves. We trust that, like seasoned craftsmen, as clinicians hone their skills at using these methods, they will become "second nature," contributing to a well-stocked and versatile toolkit for facilitating the work of adaptive change.

15

AUTOBIOGRAPHY OF THE PROBLEM

Clients for Whom the Tool Is Appropriate

Adults and adolescents with at least average literacy skills (including clients and family members), but younger children with good literacy skills could also complete the task. This tool may be used to facilitate or extend the use of externalizing language related to the problem (see Chapter 2 for a discussion of externalizing), and, therefore, may be particularly helpful with clients who are struggling with a self-image that is dominated by the problem or, conversely, with clients who have tried to ignore the problem's influence in their life. The tool would not be recommended for use with clients with expressive aphasia, agraphia, significant language impairment, or literacy skills that may not be sufficiently advanced to complete the task. Clients with cognitive impairment may also have difficulty with the complexity of the creative writing involved in the tool.

Materials Needed

Basic writing implements if writing by hand, or a computer or tablet if word processing is preferred. Alternatively, a recording device such as a tape recorder, digital recorder, or phone could be used to make an audio or video recording of a client's response that could be transcribed.

Description

This tool is designed to encourage clients to look at the problem, and their relationship with the problem, in a different way. The task for the client is to consider the problem purely from *the problem's* perspective, personifying it as a means of doing so. Clients are instructed to write an autobiography that reflects specifically on *the problem's* relationship with them, as per the instructions in Table 15–1.

Clients will typically require time to think about the task and plan out their response. Consequently, this tool is best used as a homework task that clients take away, rather than something completed within the therapy room. Of course, once it is written, the autobiography must be reviewed with the client, perhaps over multiple sessions, to examine aspects of the problem's story such as, what the problem said about the relationship, what vulnerabilities it sees in the client, when it feels the strongest, and what it fears. Exploring these types of issues with the client can lead to very fruit-

Table 15–1. Instructions for Writing the Autobiography of the Problem.

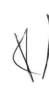

Write an autobiography from the perspective of *the problem*. Write it in the first person (i.e., using I, my, etc.) as if it were *the problem* who was doing the talking. You may wish to include topics such as why *the problem* first chose to visit you, what it wanted from you, how its demands on you changed over time, why and how it became so powerful, why it stayed around so long, what things it took from you, and what things it gave you. You may also like to consider such questions as, "Does it like you?," "How does it feed off you?," "When and where were/are its favorite places/times to try to dominate you?," and "How does it affect your relationships with other people?" For example, you might start by saying, "The thing that first attracted me to (your name) was . . ."

ful "counseling-type" conversations that start the client thinking differently about the difficulty for which they are consulting.

Case Example

Sara is a 22-year-old college student who was seeking therapy for a life-long problem with stuttering. She'd had many negative experiences related to stuttering and her self-image was completely dominated by stuttering. She struggled with alcohol and prescription drug abuse as a way of hiding from the specter of stuttering, which only served to reinforce her belief of herself as being weak and helpless. Consequently, the behavioral techniques to control stuttering that Sara had learned at a residential fluency-shaping program were, essentially, useless, as she could never apply them when she was consumed by her fear.

In our early sessions together, we discussed the possibility of thinking and talking about stuttering as an entity outside of her, as something that we could tackle together rather than either one of us trying to take on by ourselves. We agreed to call the problem *"Stuttering"* and to try to use externalizing language as much as possible both in and out of the therapy room. Sara found that she liked this idea and became quite good at talking about Stuttering in this way. After a couple of sessions of using externalizing language, Sara was invited to give Stuttering a voice by writing his (she decided Stuttering was male) autobiography. The following is Stuttering's autobiography, as written by Sara:

> *I have always been with Sara. Probably so far back that she was too young to know I was there, but I was, lurking. She did not become conscious of me until other people started pointing me out, telling her there was a right way to say things and that she was doing it wrong. She didn't know why I was giving her trouble. One night when she was seven, eight years old, her dad was tucking her into bed. As he walked down the dark hallway he said, "Goodnight, Sara." What came of her response was, "G-g-g-ggoodnight."*

Her dad stopped walking and said, "What?" in a tone that sounded like she should know better. It was times like these that Sara started to feel like I wasn't making things right, and I shouldn't be with her. Likewise, on another occasion when her older sister mocked her and she realized what I was making her sound like. I made her feel dumb and ashamed. From this point on, Sara tried to push me away. She realized I was her weakness and that letting other people discover me came at a social cost.

Being Stuttering, I want nothing more than to hold Sara back. I am her reminder of who she is. When she tries to take control, I am her refuge when she comes back in despair. I keep her safe. She does not ever have to grow or explore unknown territory as long as I am with her. With me, she knows who she is, and there is comfort for her in that. She hates me and gets depressed that I exist, but overall I think she appreciates me. When she is challenged in life, she can use me as her excuse to run and hide. I am her measure of herself; I let her know what kinds of people will be accepting of her. I choose her friends. I tell her who she can date. With Tom, I made her settle for less by telling her that was what she deserved. And for a time she believed me. For one year, I made her waste her time with him, deny her potential, and engage in destructive behavior. I also decide what kind of job/career she will work, and her potential in that. While other people around her in her company are promoted and being given bigger responsibilities, I keep her down, and I love it! She is embarrassed and ashamed of staying in the same place, but she always goes back to appreciating me, because at least with me she can give an excuse to other people, so she doesn't feel as pathetic.

Sara has plans to get rid of me. More and more each day she knows she deserves better. I feel threatened. I feel her desire to ignore me growing stronger and stronger each day. For one, she lets people know I exist, most of the time anyway. The only thing I have left to hold onto are those times when Sara loses her confident edge and decides to crawl back to me for safety. These are times that she does not want people to know about me. I can use this to maintain my power. As long as Sara doesn't like me, I have a chance.

I have humiliated her and made her feel worthless many times. As long as I can keep this up, we will be enemies forever. My plan for Sara: I don't want to lessen my grip on her until she takes her last breath. Then I have won!

Clearly, this activity highlighted many different aspects of the stuttering problem for Sara. Most profoundly, it provided a voice for *Stuttering* so that Sara could, perhaps for the first time, come face-to-face with her tormentor and begin in a sense to "talk back" to it. Sara's comments following our discussion of this tool focused on the realization that *Stuttering* was never going to stop while she continued to use it as an excuse and hide from the world; it made her face that, at times, her relationship with Stuttering was not all negative. Her renewed resolve to tackle the problem led her to taking more personal responsibility for her life, including her role in stuttering therapy, and, eventually, to stop hiding from *Stuttering* through substance abuse.

Concluding Thoughts

The intent of this approach, to reflect deeply on the problem and depict its history and implications, is compatible with basic research which demonstrates that persons who stutter (and presumably people with other communication disorders as well) actually have access to a richer, more "cognitively complex" view of themselves *with* the problem than *without* it (DiLollo, Manning, & Neimeyer, 2005). The idea of personifying the problem by writing about its effects both honors this "expertise" and encourages a new and less self-critical form of perspective taking about the relationship of the person to the problem (Rowan, 2010), opening the possibility of renegotiating the terms of the relationship to reduce the problem's negative effects, just as one might take steps in the broader social world to change a troubled relationship or to distance from "bad company." Although the problem's autobiography can be constructed in written form, as with Sara, it is also possible to interview the client—in the role of the problem—about its relationship to him or her (see Chapter 22 for more details on chair work). Regardless of the approach used, the common outcomes of this autobiographical procedure include: (1) greater clarity about the role of the problem in the client's life, (2) reduced shame about the problem as a result of externalizing it, (3) enhanced motivation to resist or work on the problem from seeing its real effects, and (4) improved insight about any subtle advantages of *having* the problem that help maintain its place in the client's life. This typically provides a good starting point for later counseling.

Frequently Asked Questions

Q: What if the client seems to have a positive relationship with the problem?

A: Not all problems will have a negative relationship with the client. DiLollo, Scherz, and Neimeyer (2013) reported on two cases of foreign accent syndrome (FAS) in which both clients experienced significant positive change that they directly related to their experience of the disorder. Similarly, in a phenomenological study of stuttering treatment, Plexico, Manning, and DiLollo (2005) found a positive aspect to the relationship between persons who stutter and their stuttering, with many stating that stuttering had made them more tolerant and empathetic. In fact, it is likely that most problems will have somewhat of a mixed relationship with the client, with some aspects of the problem being difficult (e.g., sounding different, not hearing well) while others may be positive (e.g., becoming more tolerant, learning to be assertive). Often, however, the positive aspects of the relationship may remain hidden to clients as they deal with the daily difficulties that the problem creates. By completing an autobiography of the problem, clients may, for the first time, recognize the positive aspects of the relationship. These positive aspects might be explored as potential unique outcomes on which a different way of thinking about the problem might be built.

References

DiLollo, A., Manning, W. H. & Neimeyer, R. A. (2005). Cognitive complexity as a function of speaker role for adult persons who stutter. *Journal of Constructivist Psychology, 18,* 215-236.

DiLollo, A., Scherz, J., & Neimeyer, R. A. (2013). Two cases of foreign accent syndrome: Psychosocial implications. *Journal of Constructivist Psychology, 27,* 14-30.

Plexico, L., Manning, W. H., & DiLollo, A. (2005). A phenomenological understanding of successful stuttering management. *Journal of Fluency Disorders, 30,* 1-22.

Rowan, J. (2010). *Personification: Using the dialogical self in psychotherapy and counseling.* London, UK and New York, NY: Routledge.

16

THE STORY MOUNTAIN

Clients for Whom the Tool Is Appropriate

Children ages 4 to 12 and their families can benefit from this tool, whether they are consulting for assistance with audiological or speech therapy interventions. It may not be suitable for the minority of children who are reluctant to write, but even this reluctance can often be overcome by having the counselor serve as a scribe to their oral storytelling.

Materials Needed

A large whiteboard as is used in school can provide a visual aid to the process, along with colorful markers for note-taking. Alternatively, the counselor can record the child's story on a large flip chart. In either case, a photograph can be taken of the resulting production as part of the clinical record or for use as a therapeutic document (see Chapter 24).

Description

Sometimes the concept of "narrative" as discussed in the humanities or social or medical sciences comes across as a pretty abstract idea. But of course nothing could be further from the truth: from very early childhood, young people enjoy hearing and recounting stories, and the capacity to narrate experience in a coherent (if imaginative) fashion seems to develop naturally as children acquire an increasingly stable and personalized sense of self (Nelson, 2003). Communication difficulties, of course, can challenge a positive and hopeful sense of self, and indeed pose challenges to children's understanding of what is happening to them in their family, school, and social world. For this reason it is often helpful to support children in formulating a story that "makes sense" of what they are experiencing, and that casts them in the privileged role of the storyteller.

The Story Mountain (Way, 2012) provides a simple structure for doing so. Borrowing the straightforward schema for story-writing adopted in many grammar school classrooms, the clinician first draws a "mountain" in the shape of a bell-shaped curve, dividing it into three parts corresponding to the story's beginning, middle, and end. In the presence of the child and family, the clinician then talks simply about how we all watch stories on TV, read stories in books, and tell stories about the events of our day. This can be followed by an enjoyable conversation about the kinds of stories the child likes—perhaps from a fairy tale, cartoon, television show, or book featuring a favorite character—any episode of which can be described in Story Mountain terms. For example, the *Wizard of Oz* begins with a tornado in Kansas that carries Dorothy and her little dog Toto to the magical land of Oz, where she makes friends with a Scarecrow, Lion, and Tin Man to meet the Wizard and overcome the Wicked Witch of the West, before the story ends with her returning home and awakening in her own bed. Of course this basic sketch can be fleshed out with other memorable episodes situated within it: encountering the Munchkins, setting out on the Yellow Brick Road, entering the Emerald City, being set upon by Flying Monkeys, and so forth. Just as this story suggests, beginnings give the "back story" of the action, whereas the middle usually presents a problem, challenge, or journey that the protagonist confronts, before the story ends with its resolution.

A similar narrative structure, of course, can be discerned in clinical problems centering on "dominant narratives" of communication disorder. Recognizing this, the counselor can ask the child what is happening now that is difficult—perhaps he is being teased by friends for a certain way of talking, or having trouble hearing in the classroom. Often it is this middle, problem-saturated story that is most accessible to both the child and family, as it is, after all, the reason for their consultation. As the counselor inquires about it and the young child recounts examples of what is happening now, the counselor briefly notes these in a few phrases on the middle section of the Story Mountain, giving the child's story priority, but also asking him or her if it would be okay to get the parent's ideas about this part of the story as well. These can then be added briefly, perhaps in a different color of marker, but only if the child gives assent to each addition. Continuing in this way, the family can readily reconstruct the current challenges faced by the child, while conveying his or her central role as storyteller or editor of the account—a very different stance than someone simply subjugated to the problem. Alternatively, older children who enjoy writing might be encouraged to make notes about the storytelling conversation on the Story Mountain drawing, adding notes about their parents' contributions, and then writing up the story as a flowing whole to help integrate it more fully. In either case, the child is encouraged to master the story—to make it one that he authors, rather than one that "authors" him.

Next, the counselor can turn to the beginning of the story, of the child's and family's life before the problem entered the scene. Here, children can sometimes have trouble remembering the "good times" that came before, especially when the problem was gradual, congenital, or of long standing. But even in such cases, parents can often relate with pride stories of the child's birth, their love for the new baby, funny accounts, perhaps half-remembered by the child, and so on, prompted toward specific, concrete stories by the counselor's curiosity. As each bit is contributed, the child is invited to elaborate, agree, or disagree as the counselor or child makes brief notes on the rising curve of the Story Mountain's ascending slope, to the point that the problem was first detected or addressed. Typically this beginning chapter of the story provides a strong testament to the family's love and solidarity, countering in some measure their sense of powerlessness in relation to the problem.

Finally, the counselor turns attention to the end of the story, which might begin with the treatment now being received, and lead imaginatively into what the hoped-for future might look like, being led once again by the child's sense of what might constitute a "happy ending," but also including the parents' and counselor's ideas about how the child and family might cope with the challenges the problem poses, now and in the future. The goal here is to evoke a preferred story of communication competence and connection to counter the dominant narrative of disability, perhaps drawing on the unique qualities of the child that can be discerned in the beginning chapter of the story, but that have sometimes been eclipsed in the problematic middle. This work can benefit from using *externalization* of the problem (such as the lisp, stuttering, or hearing problem) as an opponent or mischievous companion throughout the conversation, but the Story Mountain can also be used to tell the tale without this embellishment. In either case, the idea is to help the child and family to author a fuller account of the child's life before and beyond the problem, conferring on the child the more empowered role of storyteller and editor.

Case Example

When Ronnie, age 8, and his parents came to the clinic, they seemed defeated and discouraged. Ronnie had been stuttering for over 4 years now, and his parents' early hopes that he would "grow out of it" had faded. He was having trouble in school and seemed to be isolating himself and not even trying to make any friends. We had been working with Ronnie for a few sessions, trying to get him to control his disfluencies through some fluency shaping tools but also trying some desensitizing activities to help him deal with the emotional aspects of his stuttering. As Ronnie had shown interest in superheroes—his favorite movie was *The Avengers*—we had begun talking about fighting the "fear monster" and being "heroic." Ronnie appeared to like these ideas, but didn't seem to be able to cast himself in the role of the "hero" or even to feel that he was in any way in control of his own story.

In an attempt to get a better understanding of Ronnie's complete story, we engaged him in a process of story telling using the *Story Mountain*. We started out by explaining to Ronnie and his parents that stories form a big part of our lives, from the books we read, to the TV shows we watch, and even just the stories that we tell about ourselves. To get things started, we asked Ronnie to tell us about his day, starting with the morning through to now. He recounted how he had gotten out of bed, had breakfast, gone off to school, what he'd done during recess and an interesting science class, and how his Mom and Dad picked him up and brought him to the clinic. "Okay," we said, "Well, you just told us a story. You see, it had a beginning—when you woke up this morning and got ready for school; a middle—when you were at school and then coming here; and, if we continued, you could tell us about what might happen at the end of your story—like, maybe Mom and Dad take you for ice cream on the way home, you have dinner, watch TV together, and go to bed." Ronnie grinned, "I like that end."

Now that Ronnie and his parents understood the concept, we drew a basic Story Mountain on a whiteboard (Figure 16-1) and showed them how the beginning, middle, and end of the story mapped onto the picture. We told Ronnie that this was going to be *his* Story Mountain—"Mount Ronnie" we called it—and so it needed to tell his story. We started by asking Ronnie to describe what was happening now that was difficult for him. As he talked, we wrote notes on the story mountain to capture his story. Ronnie talked about how his stuttering at school was a problem and how there were a number of kids in his class who were mean and bullied him. He mentioned a particularly distressing event that happened earlier this week when a substitute teacher called on him in class to read out loud. When he refused, the teacher became angry and made him stand up and read the passage. As Ronnie tried to read and got more and more anxious, he had a severe block. Thinking he was acting out, the teacher made a remark about Ronnie not being able to read, and Ronnie began to cry. This embarrassed him severely and led to further teasing and bullying from the boys in his class. We asked Ronnie if it was okay to get Mom and Dad to tell part of the story, and he agreed. As Mom and Dad told us about

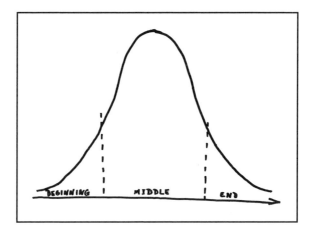

Figure 16–1. The basic Story Mountain diagram.

some of the things going on in Ronnie's life, we added them to the center of the story mountain picture (after checking with Ronnie that they were aspects of his story that he wanted to include). Mom and Dad filled in parts of Ronnie's story that focused on his isolation (which was one of their main concerns), such as quitting the soccer team, leaving summer camp, and spending a lot of time alone. To bring us up to the present time, we asked Ronnie if we could add "starting therapy" to his story mountain. He agreed and suggested that we also add "fighting the fear monster" as this was his favorite part of therapy.

Having completed the "middle" of Mount Ronnie, we worked with Ronnie and his Mom and Dad to build the beginning of the story, which started with Ronnie's birth and his early development. The family had fun talking about Ronnie as a baby and sharing stories about him with the clinicians. Mom even had a few pictures of Ronnie at various young ages on her iPhone that she shared—much to Ronnie's delight and embarrassment!

With the beginning of Ronnie's story mountain complete, we next turned to the end of the story. We started by talking about speech therapy and, in particular, the concept of "fighting the fear monster." Ronnie was able to tell Mom and Dad about how

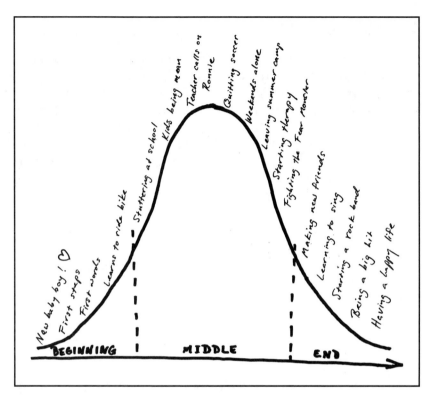

Figure 16–2. Ronnie's Story Mountain.

important strategies are when fighting a monster—"Just like Iron Man did in The Avengers," he told them. After Ronnie told his parents all about speech therapy, we asked him, "Okay, Ronnie, what might happen next? If we want to make a good ending for your story, what might that look like? Maybe Mom and Dad can help us come up with a happy ending for your story." We spent some time talking about how things might change for Ronnie in the future, rejecting some ideas and liking others. We started out with Ronnie making new friends—something that his parents were anxious for him to include. Ultimately, however, Ronnie guided what went on his story mountain, and his vision had him learning to sing and starting a successful rock band! (Figure 16-2)

Concluding Thoughts

Simple though it may be, the Story Mountain can help children address three important narrative tasks: to find a thread of continuity to the past, to organize a sometimes confusing present, and to project into a hopeful future. Moreover, by being positioned as the main authors and editors of their stories, children can gain a sense of mastery over difficult problems, and invite the collaboration of their parents in validating who they have been and where they want to go. Finally, through the inclusion of therapy as a chapter in the book of their lives, the Story Mountain gives a place of importance to the clinician's technical intervention, without making the mistake of viewing it as the entirety of the client's life story. It can in this sense offer a "container" for the whole of therapy and adaptive counseling, which might also include several of the other methods included in the Toolkit section of this book (e.g., play therapy and therapeutic documentation).

Frequently Asked Questions

Q: Some children have a hard time remembering good times before the problem. How can the counselor draw out the beginning of the story if this happens?

A: That is one of the advantages of having the parents participate in the counseling session, as the clinician can ask the child, "Could your mom and dad help us remember what life was like when you were little?" He can then turn to the parents and prompt them with questions like, "What was your earliest memory of Ronnie?" "What do you remember about some of your favorite times with him when he was a toddler?" Soon one memory will trigger another, and the child often will join in the telling once more.

Q: What if the child is very young, like 4 or 5, and can't read the words on the Story Mountain image?

A: This isn't really a problem, because the counselor can read it back when the family is done, or can use a simple drawing instead of words, like the image of a baby to represent birth, a pencil to symbolize school, or a soccer ball to depict involvement in sports.

Even if the artwork is bad, the family can have fun laughing at the counselor's attempt! Alternatively, the child can draw the picture, and can use separate sheets of numbered paper if she needs more room, with the counselor putting the numbers on the story mountain to indicate where they fall in the story. Of course, the family can brainstorm about what kind of picture could be used to represent the significant episodes in the story, but the child should be given editorial authority to decide what is included.

Q: How does the counselor integrate the Story Mountain back into more technical therapy for the disorder?

A: Once the story is recorded on the form or white board, the counselor can circle or put a star next to therapy, if the child or family inserted it into the account, or if not can place it on the downward slope at the point the problematic middle begins to change into the preferred end. She can then ask the child and family what ideas they have about how therapy can help contribute to a happy ending to the story.

References

Nelson, K. (2003). Narrative and the emergence of a consciousness of self. In G. D. Fireman, T. E. McVay, & O. J. Flanagan (Eds.), *Narrative and consciousness: Literature, psychology and the brain* (pp. 17-36). New York, NY: Oxford.

Way, P. (2012). The story mountain. In R. A. Neimeyer (Ed.), *Tools of grief therapy: Creative practices for counseling the bereaved* (pp. 196-198). New York, NY: Routledge.

17

DRAWING

Clients for Whom the Tool Is Appropriate

Children and adults of all ages (including clients and family members) can benefit from this tool. This tool may be used to facilitate or extend the use of externalizing language related to the problem (see Chapters 8 and 11 for more details about externalizing), and, therefore, may be particularly helpful with clients who are struggling with a self-image that is dominated by the problem or, conversely, with clients who have tried to ignore the problem's influence in their life. In addition, the tool may be useful with children or adults who have difficulty with tools that involve more complex verbal or written tasks, and for clients who appear reluctant to engage in conversations about the emotional aspects of their communication problem. The tool may not be suitable for clients with limited motor function who cannot hold or adequately control drawing implements.

Materials Needed

Basic drawing implements (i.e., pencils, crayons, markers, etc.) and paper are needed. Alternatively, a computer with a painting or drawing program may be used. Some clients may prefer to paint or sculpt as their form of artistic expression. These would be used in the same way as simple drawing.

Description

Drawing is a natural mode of communication that children and adults rarely resist and that offers a way to express feelings and thoughts in a way that is less threatening than strictly verbal means (Malchiodi, 2001). Drawings have been used as projective measures of personality (e.g., Oster & Montgomery, 1996) and in the evaluation of cognitive abilities in children (Silver, 2001). Working with children, Winnicott (1971) found that drawing helped increase client–clinician interaction and expanded the effectiveness and depth of the therapeutic relationship. In the field of communication disorders, drawing has been used with persons who stutter (Lev-Wiesel, Shabat, & Tsur, 2005; McCormack, 2013; Stewart & Brosh, 1997) and as an alternative form of communication for persons with severe aphasia (e.g., Morgan & Helm-Estabrooks, 1987).

This tool is designed to help clients reflect on the problem in ways that might be different from their regular verbal descriptions of the problem and its impact in their life. Often, certain images or feelings can be difficult to put into words. Creative endeavors such as drawing or painting can sometimes provide a means for expression that allows a more complete portrayal of feelings. For using this tool, two drawing activities are suggested to provide clients with an opportunity to contrast images and feelings related to their relationship with the problem that may otherwise be difficult to express. A comparison and discussion of these drawings may help clinicians and clients identify potential iMoments that might have been otherwise difficult to uncover verbally. Clients should be instructed to not be concerned with the "quality" of their drawings, as even the simplest drawing can have very powerful and meaningful implications to the artist. Table 17–1 shows the instructions that are provided to the client.

After completing their drawings, clients should be encouraged to explain the drawings to the clinician, telling the story of each drawing. Following this, clients can be invited to reflect on how

Table 17–1. Instructions for Drawing Activity

Note: Do not be concerned with the quality of your drawing. You can draw whatever comes to mind (i.e., it does not have to be a picture of a person) and you can use whatever implements and/or media that are available. Allow yourself to be creative.

1. Draw a picture of yourself with your companion, *the Problem*.

2. Draw a picture of yourself without *the Problem* as your companion.

Table 17–2. Questions for Clients About Their Drawings

1. How are these two drawings different?

2. Do you look or act differently in the two drawings?

3. If so, what might this mean to you?

4. Which one of these drawings most accurately depicts the "real" you?

5. Do you have a preference for either of the drawings?

6. If you could add something to one of the drawings, what would it be?

the two drawings are different. Table 17–2 lists a series of questions that clinicians might ask clients to help identify possible iMoments.

Case Example

Ben was a 37-year-old male who stutters. He had received a lot of speech therapy during his life but continued to struggle with disfluencies and varying levels of anxiety and avoidance. During one of his sessions, we talked about doing a drawing activity to help him try to begin to look at stuttering in a different way. He decided that he would work on his drawings at home, so I gave him the simple instructions shown in Table 17–1.

Ben made the unusual choice of completing the drawings, shown in Figures 17–1 and 17–2, on his computer using a "Paint" program. His drawings depicted a scene rather than a person— also rather unusual, as most people, given instructions to draw

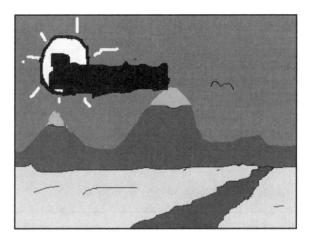

Figure 17–1. Ben's drawing of himself with stuttering.

themselves, draw a person. I asked Ben to walk me though his pictures. He described the first picture (Figure 17-1), representing him with stuttering, pointing out that stuttering was the black cloud that partially blots out the sun. He also pointed out that he was the bird—alone in the sky, and that the river running off into the distance represents his life. He described the second picture (Figure 17-2) as being exactly the same as the first, but now stuttering is gone, the sun is shining, and other birds have joined him in the sky. I asked Ben to tell me about how he was different in the two pictures. He said that, in the first picture, under the influence of stuttering, he didn't attract other birds, but with stuttering gone, other birds came to fly with him. "That's interesting," I said, "I wonder how that worked . . . because the only difference between the two pictures is that the stuttering cloud has gone. It doesn't look like the bird has changed." Ben thought for a while. "I see what you mean. Its kind of like it was the cloud that kept the other birds away, but that doesn't really make sense. So, if it wasn't the cloud it must have been the bird . . . me!" I hoped that he would explore this line of thinking further, so I asked, "I wonder what changed for the bird between the first and second pictures." He responded,

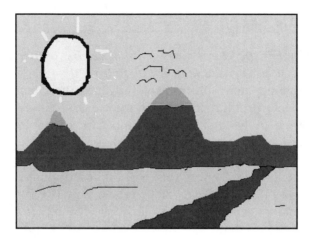

Figure 17–2. Ben's drawing of himself without stuttering.

"I guess he is more confident and outgoing in the second picture, and that is what attracts the other birds." I recognized a possible *reconceptualization iMoment* in this conversation, so I asked, "I wonder how he made that change . . . and why he wasn't like that in the first picture just because there was a cloud in the sky?"

Ben and I continued this conversation over the course of several sessions, eventually leading to a reconceptualization that it wasn't stuttering that was holding him back and that he could make the changes that he wanted regardless of whether his speech was fluent or not.

Concluding Thoughts

As a creative act, drawing will sometimes lead to insights that verbal exchanges cannot access. In many cases, too, clients' drawings will be relatively abstract, allowing a form of *projection* to occur when client and clinician start trying to understand what the drawing might mean.

Frequently Asked Questions

Q: What if the client cannot interpret his or her drawing? What if all he or she sees is just a drawing?

A: Drawings may still be useful, even if the client lacks the capacity to interpret the drawing. In these cases, clinicians and significant others in the client's life might be able to draw some tentative conclusions from the images. In addition, drawing can be used to identify constructs that clients have in relation to certain topics or domains, in a similar way that written descriptions are used in Crockett's (1965) *Role Category Questionnaire* (RCQ) to identify interpersonal constructs. For example, we recently worked with a teenager with high-functioning autism and used drawing as one way to elicit constructs about people and about the future that he sees for himself.

Q: Is it okay for clients to keep the drawings they do in therapy?

A: The drawings belong to the client, so they can do with them as they please. I always ask clients if I can make a copy of any drawings (and other material) that they produce in sessions. If a particular drawing seems to impact a client, I will suggest he or she keep the drawing and mount it on a wall at home and refer to it and replay the conversations that we had about it. In this way, the drawing may act as a type of *therapeutic document* (see Chapter 24).

References

Crockett, W. H. (1965). Cognitive complexity and impression formation. In B. A. Maher (Ed.), *Progress in experimental personality research* (Vol. 2, pp. 47–90). New York, NY: Academic Press.

Lev-Wiesel, R., Shabat, A., & Tsur, A. (2005). Stuttering as reflected in adults' self-figure drawings. *Journal of Developmental and Physical Disabilities, 17*, 85–93.

Malchiodi C. A. (2001). Using drawing as intervention with traumatized children. *Trauma and Loss: Research and Interventions, 1*, 11–19.

McCormack, J. (2011). *The experience of people who stutter in a therapy programme using art* (Master's thesis). Dublin City University, Dublin, Ireland.

Morgan, A. L. R., & Helm-Estabrooks, N. (1987). Back to the drawing board: A treatment program for nonverbal aphasic patients. *Clinical Aphasiology, 17*, 64–72.

Oster, G., & Montgomery, S. (1996). *Clinical uses of drawings.* Northvale, NJ: Jason Aronson.

Silver, R. (2001). *Art as language.* Philadelphia, PA: Brunner-Routledge.

Stewart, T., & Brosh, H. (1997). The use of drawings in the management of adults who stammer. *Journal of Fluency Disorders, 22*, 35–50.

Winnicott, D. (1971). *Playing and reality.* New York, NY: Basic Books

18

DEAR JOHN LETTER

Clients for Whom the Tool Is Appropriate

Adults and adolescents with at least average literacy skills (including clients and family members) can use this tool. Younger children with good literacy skills could also complete the task, although in these cases it might be framed as a "letter to a friend you are not going to see anymore" or a "letter to a bully you finally stood up to." This tool would typically be used after clients have made progress toward an alternative narrative that resists the influence of *the problem.* In this way it can be helpful as an early retelling of such stories of resistance, with printed copies also serving as *therapeutic documents* (see Chapter 24) that can be read and re-read to reinforce the emerging story. The tool would not be recommended for use with clients with expressive aphasia, agraphia, significant language impairment, or literacy skills that may not be sufficiently advanced to complete the task. Clients with cognitive impairment may also have difficulty with the complexity of the creative writing involved in the tool.

Materials Needed

Basic writing implements will be needed if this is to be handwritten; a computer or tablet will be needed if word processing is preferred. The letter can be also be in the form of an e-mail or a posting on the client's home page on a social network site such as Facebook.

Description

This tool is designed to encourage clients to look at the problem, and their relationship with the problem, in a different way. It is based on the concept of externalizing (White & Epston, 1990) that we discussed in Chapters 6, 8, and 10, that encourages clients to objectify and personify the problem to allow greater focus, feeling of control, and resistance to the problem's influence. The task for clients writing the Dear John letter, therefore, is to consider the problem as separate from themselves but still in relationship with them. A key feature of the Dear John Letter is that the client expresses in writing his or her resistance to the influence of *the Problem* and projects a future that is free from its dominance. By doing this, clients may provide clues to potential iMoments that have been lost over time or which went previously unrecognized. The instructions provided to the client appear in Table 18-1.

Table 18–1. Instructions for Writing the Dear John Letter

It is likely that *the Problem* has been your "companion" for a long period of time. Sometimes it is difficult to break away from long-term relationships, as our lives with the other seem to be so intricately intertwined, both socially and emotionally. This may apply to your relationship with *the Problem.*

One way of "breaking off" a relationship when you cannot speak to the partner face-to-face may be to write a letter—a "Dear John" letter as they have become known—that expresses your feelings about the relationship and the circumstances that have led you to seek to end or change that relationship at that particular time. In this exercise, write a "Dear John" letter to *the Problem*, talking to it about both the positive and negative aspects of your relationship with it, why you are currently engaged in trying to remove yourself from, or change, that relationship, and the plans you have for the future of the relationship and for your future outside of the relationship.

Case Example

Ashley, a 17-year-old girl who stutters, had been in therapy many times throughout her life. She had learned both fluency shaping and stuttering modification skills and could, almost effortlessly, produce an easy onset, cancellation, or pull out on command. What she had always struggled with, however, was standing up to *Stuttering's* influence. She believed *Stuttering* when it told her she couldn't go to Prom; she gave in to *Stuttering's* insistence that she should be ashamed of the way she speaks; and she allowed *Stuttering* to bully her into believing that it would always hold the upper hand. These were some of the externalizing ways that we talked about stuttering as Ashley tried to take back control of her life. As Ashley grew more and more comfortable thinking and talking about stuttering in this way, it helped her to begin to view her relationship with *Stuttering* differently—to begin to take a stance against *Stuttering's* influence and to then be more effective using the technical skills that she had learned over her many years of speech therapy. As we came toward the end of our work together, Ashley wrote the following "Dear John letter" to *Stuttering*:

> *Dear Stuttering,*
>
> *Hello. I guess I don't have to introduce myself because we know each other quite well. I think that you arrived at my house in second grade. You might've been there long before but maybe you were hidden in a way, because my parents just thought I was learning to talk or something.*
>
> *Sometimes I have tried to hide you, believe it or not, and I still do. But instead of a game of hide and seek, you don't hide willingly. It's not like I can say: 'Yo, stuttering! Get lost for a while, okay? I have been trying hard to deal with you and not try to hide you but it is tough!'*
>
> *As you know, I have been trying to avoid you, and I'm sorry for that. You have come into my life and I think you are here to stay. Even though I can control you with stretching, slowing down, and so forth, you will still always be there, sneaking up in bad situations. Now, I know it's not your fault; it's not really mine either.*

I just have to work on not tensing up and using my techniques. My techniques make the stuttering come out easier. So, instead of things like: b-bb-bbbbb-bbbb-all. I'd say: b-b-ball. But, I think you know what I am talking about. Am I right? It's also hard to talk about you with other people, and I guess that is relating to hiding you. I mean, what am I going to do, just go up to one of my friends and say: Guess what? I stutter, but you probably already know. I mean sometimes it is easier than others. If a friend says something like: Oh, what are you doing this afternoon? Instead of saying: Oh, nothing, I'll say: Well, I have a speech therapy appointment. And then that might lead to a longer conversation. I think the difficult thing is to just start the conversation, because it is hard to come up with that first sentence. Do you know what I mean? But, once I am in the conversation I am totally fine and I am almost as relaxed as in other conversations. Almost. I think the one good thing about you is that you have helped me be more understanding. Now, understanding is a pretty broad word. I mean if someone has a lisp, and everyone is making fun of him or her sometimes I may stand up for that person, because people really have no reason to make fun of him or her.

It is hard to explain but I just feel more compassion for people, if you know what I mean.

Well, Stuttering, I think it's time for me to wrap this letter up. I think I have said what I need to say. I think that I am getting much better about being open with you. And I have tried to not avoid you as much but, I have to admit, I don't willingly tell people I stutter. Normally at the end of a letter, I would say something like: Hope to see you soon, but in this case, it is more like: Hope to not see you soon. But, I think if we run into each other, which I am positive we will, I will do just fine, and just have to deal with your company.

Love,

Ashley

After writing the letter, Ashley read it aloud to me and we talked about what it was like to take the stance of resisting *Stuttering* and, essentially, breaking off the relationship. She said that it was a little "scary" because *Stuttering* had been her companion for a long time. She knew that she wasn't getting rid of *Stuttering* totally, and actually took some comfort in that, but she also said that she knew that *Stuttering* would never again have the power that it used to have in her life. Ashley indicated that she intended to keep this letter with her and read it frequently to remind her that she was the one in control.

Concluding Thoughts

As a flexible technique, the Dear John letter can have many purposes: to document the negative influence of the communication disorder on the client, to claim more voice in the relationship, to relate to the problem more on the client's terms, or to assert the intent to end the relationship altogether. Often, as in Ashley's case, the client expresses some ambivalence in the relationship, like renegotiating future engagements with a familiar companion one has outgrown. Writing such a letter and reading it to the counselor can both be empowering steps, and can provide a kind of container or framework for much of their technical and adaptive work together, which can help the client win back more control from the communication problem and its real effects in the social world.

Frequently Asked Questions

Q: Does the Dear John letter have to reflect a complete removal of the problem from the person's life?

A: No. The goal for the Dear John letter is for it to reflect the emerging story of resistance to the influence of the problem. In some cases, this might actually mean a complete "breaking off" of the relationship with the problem. In many cases, however, as in the case example above, the problem will remain in the person's life in some form; the key in these cases is for the person to construct a preferred story of resistance to the influence of the problem.

Reference

White, M., & Epston, D. (1990). *Narrative means to therapeutic ends.* New York, NY: W.W. Norton and Company.

19

THE DOWNWARD ARROW

Clients for Whom the Tool Is Appropriate

This tool is appropriate for adult and adolescent clients who experience a sudden downturn in mood or a spike of anxiety in connection with a stressful event related to their communication or swallowing disorder, and are interested in learning more about the silent assumptions being triggered by the event. The tool would not be recommended for someone with significant cognitive impairment that interferes with introspection or that produces expressive aphasia, as well as for children under the age of 12 who are unaccustomed to "thinking about thinking."

Materials Needed

A clipboard, writing tablet, and pen are all that is required to visually depict the downward arrow elicited from a client in the course of an interview. The resulting diagram can then be saved for the clinical record, or (copied and) given to the client for further reflection and therapeutic homework.

Description

Virtually every client contending with a communication disorder is familiar with those moments when they encounter an impasse or setback—a hearing aid works poorly in the din of a crowded restaurant, a speech disfluency raises visible discomfort in a listener, an attempt to find the right word draws a blank and produces an awkward silence. Similarly, most clients experience moments when they suffer some level of "social penalty" related to their communication disorder: a group conversation moves on without waiting for the person who stutters to give his opinion, a teenage girl with a severe hearing loss is labeled a "freak" by some classmates because they have to use a microphone and FM system in their small group discussions at school. When this happens, clients can "catastrophize" (Burns, 1999), experiencing a cascade of depressive or anxiety-arousing thoughts that quickly deflate their sense of self-esteem or magnify their fears, and that unfold so rapidly and involuntarily that cognitive therapists call them *automatic thoughts*.

How can a clinician help a client put the brakes on this process? The first step is to capture the thoughts on paper so that they can be recognized and examined more closely. From a constructivist standpoint, the *downward arrow* represents a convenient tool for doing just that, making the implicit explicit in the form of a simple diagram that traces the deeper (and often hidden) implications of the client's catastrophic thinking (Neimeyer, 1993). For example, a man with partial hearing loss that followed a viral infection that damaged his auditory nerve might shake his head sadly in talking about his "failed attempt" to accompany his wife to a musical concert, during which he repeatedly experienced acute discomfort when she and others around him would clap explosively following the stirring performance of a piece. Inquiring about what troubled him about this, the client might note that he felt that people would see him as a "fool" for putting his fingers in his ears to dampen the pain of the applause. Using the downward arrow, the clinician might then simply ask, "Suppose that were true, that people really were thinking you were a fool for plugging your ears during the applause; what would that mean to you?" The man might reply, "They'd think I hated the music, and had no business being there."

Noting this on paper and continuing this cycle of recursive questioning, the clinician might then again ask, "Okay, let's assume that were true, that they really did think you hated the performance and shouldn't be there. What would that mean to you?" The client could respond, "I should just leave, and maybe wait in the lobby for my wife." Repeated questioning presupposing the truth of each statement might continue to trace the client's line of emotional reasoning, perhaps revealing fatalistic conclusions that the world of music that was once a great joy to him is now off limits, that he is on his way to total deafness, or even that he is no longer a fitting husband and companion for his wife, but only fit to live the life of a recluse. As the interview unfolds over the course of a few minutes, the clinician simply writes down each of these conclusions in a series (usually with four or five steps) without immediately disputing them, with a downward arrow indicating each. Showing the series to the client, the clinician can help him see where his automatic thoughts are taking him, and the two together can begin to consider whether the chain reaction leading to his sense of deflation, embarrassment, and despair is the only possible way of viewing the event (i.e., maybe there are "alternative ways of construing" the events), and whether there are any ways to "break the chain" through more adaptive thinking or behavior. Once clearly visualized, the downward spiral can seem far less compelling, and clients commonly often begin to dispute their implicit conclusions spontaneously, with minimal prompting by the counselor. In contrast, as long as the landslide of catastrophic thinking remains largely unconscious, it can continue to work its hidden effects on our clients' mood, and trigger all manner of avoidance behaviors that reinforce the dominant narrative of their "brokenness."

Case Example

"I don't think I can do this," said Amy, a normally cheerful, outgoing, 20-year-old self-described "tomboy." She was in speech therapy to get treatment for recurring vocal nodules brought on by vocal abuse and poor vocal hygiene. Amy was learning to use a less intense, breathy voice and to avoid the loud, smoky environments that she and her friends often frequented. As she arrived for this session, I could tell that Amy was struggling with something as she was subdued and perhaps even a little depressed. "What's going on?" I asked. "Its my friends," she said, in a voice that I could tell had been "abused" recently. "They just don't seem to care. They know that I can't go to *Kirby's* (the local club that they frequented) but last night they wouldn't change their plans, even though I explained to them that I shouldn't go. . . . It was, like, 'Either come to Kirby's with us or stay home.'" I waited, "So . . . I went . . . and now my voice is bad again."

This event with her friends had Amy much more upset than I would have expected, so I suspected that maybe there was more going on than just not sticking to her treatment plan. I said to Amy, "What's got you so upset by this?" "I don't know," she replied, "I am just so mad at my friends! They just don't seem to care about what it is I am trying to do . . . All they care about is going out and having a good time!" I said, "Well, lets talk about this. Maybe we can try something that might help you to understand where these feelings are coming from . . . because while you are so upset like this, its going to be hard for you to stick with what we are trying to do to improve your voice."

Amy agreed, so I asked her, "You said that your friends just don't seem to care about what it is that you are trying to do. Suppose that were true, that your friends really don't care about what you are trying to do; what would that mean to you?" She replied, "Then they really don't care about me!" I wrote this down under the first statement, connecting the two statements with an arrow (Figure 19–1). "Okay, lets assume that were true, that your friends really don't care about you; what would that mean to you?" This time, Amy took a little longer, "That I don't really have any friends, I guess." Again, I wrote this under the other statements and connected them with an arrow. "Lets suppose that also were true, that you don't really have any friends; what would that mean to you?" Amy took even longer to respond this time. With tears in her eyes, she looked at me and said, "That I am not very likeable; a loser!" Amy's history included frequent geographic relocations during her childhood, and struggles with weight gain and frequent feelings of isolation in her high-school years, and it seemed as if the behavior

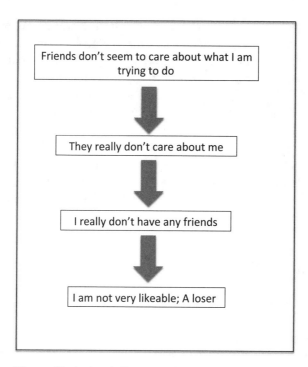

Figure 19–1. Amy's Downward Arrow diagram.

of her friends had unwittingly triggered a vulnerability to these old, familiar feelings. Consequently, this seemed like an appropriate point at which to stop the downward arrow questions, so I wrote this last statement under the others and, again, connected it with an arrow. I showed the downward arrow sketch (Figure 19-1) to Amy and gave her time to take in the visual of the spiral that her automatic thoughts were leading her down.

After a while, I asked Amy if she had any comments. She stayed silent for a while, then looked at me and said, "I'm not a loser." Although tempted to reinforce her positive statement by agreeing with it, I instead asked, "Tell me what makes you say that." Amy described a number of positive attributes that she identified with and, this time, I did repeat these aspects of her preferred identity back to her. Following this, I directed her attention back to the downward arrow sketch and asked, "So, given what you have just told me about yourself, are there alternative ways that we could interpret what happened with your friends?" Without a lot of thought, Amy replied, "I think maybe they just don't really understand how important it is to me to fix my voice. I mean, Josh even told me that he thinks my old voice is 'sexy' and he doesn't think I should change it! They don't really get that there is something bad going on with my vocal folds and that it will only get worse if I don't do something about it now."

Following this, Amy and I discussed how she might talk with her friends about how important it was to her to take care of her voice, what that was going to take, and how she was going to need their help to succeed.

Concluding Thoughts

Sigmund Freud once famously remarked that dreams were the "royal road to the unconscious," meaning that teasing out the significance of our nighttime dreams could open the door to a deeper understanding of the person's implicit emotional life. In a certain sense, the *downward arrow* represents another road to these unconscious associations—perhaps not as scenic as Freud's, but possibly more direct and efficient! When driven by a sensitive and empathic clinician, the downward arrow method can even be something of an "interstate highway" leading directly into the heart of those concerns triggered by a troubling event, in a way that opens it to closer inspection and deconstruction.

As clinicians gain experience with this simple method, they can begin to weave it naturally into conversation, perhaps even beyond the clinical context. For example, one of our audiology students, after reading about and experimenting with the downward arrow tool, spoke about using it with a friend to process troubling experiences in their own lives: "Using the *downward arrow*, we really get down to the deep reasons why some of the experiences we have bother us so much. By doing this, we remove some of the control the experience has over us and we regain an ownership of sorts. If we were to let every negative incident rule our lives, we'd end up living a very unconscious life; we'd be going through the motions, letting life happen to us, rather than making things happen in our lives. This *downward arrow* technique serves to detach inappropriate meaning from events that need not dominate our lives." It would be hard to state the deeper intent of the method more eloquently than this.

Frequently Asked Questions

Q: What if our client's initial thoughts are valid, that they really do have a communication problem, or that people are evaluating them negatively? How can it be useful to make them even more aware of how bad this makes them feel?

A: This is a good question, as the starting point for the downward arrow usually is a realistic thought about a concrete situation the client experienced. But what commonly happens when this triggers a strong emotional reaction for the client is that he or she experiences a cognitive avalanche of negative or alarming conclusions that follow on this, which quickly become more generalized and unrealistic. By capturing this often unrecognized process on paper, the downward arrow makes it much more conscious, giving the client and counselor a chance to question these conclusions, and where valid, consider how to respond to them more adaptively.

Q: Okay, but how does this fit into the technical work of treating clients, whether getting them to wear a hearing aid, coaching them in communication skills, or modifying their speech or swallowing behavior? Doesn't this get off track from the necessary work of improving their communication?

A: Actually, like most of the tools addressed in this section of the book, the downward arrow helps get the client back *on track* with technical interventions. This is because setbacks are nearly inevitable in all treatments, and unexamined and unsupported, they can contribute to a client's discouragement or fear, and lead to avoidance of necessary practice or even discontinuation of therapy. As the downward arrow commonly takes only five minutes to elicit and another few minutes to process, it can efficiently help reinforce the client's resourcefulness in coping with future obstacles and restore the momentum of therapy.

References

Burns, D. (1999). *The feeling good handbook.* New York, NY: Penguin.

Neimeyer, R. A. (1993). Constructivist approaches to the measurement of meaning. In G. J. Neimeyer (Ed.), *Constructivist assessment: A casebook* (pp. 58–103). Newbury Park, CA: Sage.

20

SELF-CHARACTERIZATION

Robert A. Neimeyer, Chris Constantino, and Anthony DiLollo

Clients for Whom the Tool Is Appropriate

This tool is appropriate for adults and adolescents (including clients and family members) with at least average literacy skills, but younger children with good literacy skills could also complete the task. The tool would not be recommended for use with clients with expressive aphasia, agraphia, significant language impairment, or literacy skills that may not be sufficiently advanced to complete the task. Clients with cognitive impairment may also have difficulty with the complexity of the creative writing involved in the tool. However, even in some of these cases, use of dictation software could allow many of these clients to complete the writing without difficulty.

Materials Needed

Basic writing implements are need if this is going to be handwritten, or a computer, tablet, or recording device if word processing or dictation is preferred.

Description

As we have seen, one theme that runs through narrative constructivist psychology concerns the nature of the self, that is, our sense of ourselves as having a personal identity, grounded in a life story that is uniquely our own. While not denying genetic contributions to our personality, constructivists emphasize the significant extent to which "we make ourselves up as we go along," drawing on the discourses and practices of our place and time. While different theorists emphasize the personal, social, or cultural basis of identity, all would agree that who we are is an expression of those particular values, goals, and relationships that emerge from our unique "positioning" in the larger meaning systems of our families, societies and historical periods. In practical terms, this helps us appreciate the distinctive contributions of our clients' personal and cultural frameworks to both the problems they present, and to their solution.

But how can we hope to gain insight into something as abstract as our clients' "identities," especially given the technical demands of our work with communication disorders? One radical idea advanced by the psychologist George Kelly nearly 60 years ago was to simply ask them! Of course, stated abstractly the question can seem daunting, if not downright strange. But phrased playfully, in the language of make-believe as a homework assignment, it can be surprisingly feasible for the client, as well as illuminating for the professional. With minor modification, Kelly's (1955) original instructions, printed on an otherwise blank sheet of paper, appear in Table 20–1.

Several features of this simple instruction are worth noting (Kelly, 1955). First, it requests that clients offer a "sketch" of who they are, rather than a carefully worked out, comprehensive and

Table 20–1. Instructions for the Self-Characterization Technique

I want you to write a character sketch of _____, just as if (he or she) were the principal character in a play, book, movie, or television show. Write it as it might be written by a friend who knew (him or her) very *intimately* and very *sympathetically*, perhaps better than anyone ever really could know (him or her). Be sure to write it in third person. For example, start out by saying, _____ is . . .

documented "analysis" of their personality. Second, rather than adopting a "pathologizing" framework that focuses on psychological, medical, or behavioral problems or disorders, it encourages the client to see him- or herself as a character in a story read, told or performed, and to do so basically from the standpoint of a sympathetic "best friend." This feature of the instructions goes some distance toward softening many clients' tendency toward self-criticism, subtly countering the hopelessness that undermines any attempt at self-change, and instead helps reveal clients' hidden resources and longer range goals, both of which can be enlisted in the service of therapeutic objectives. Third, the instructions encourage the client to take a third person perspective, speaking in terms of "he" or "she," rather than "I." The wisdom of this linguistic shift is supported by recent research that indicates that writing about oneself in a "self-distancing" rather than "self-immersed" fashion carries many benefits, lightening the burden of negative and self-evaluative emotions, increasing hopefulness, and improving one's problem solving (Kross & Ayduk, 2010). In short, these simple instructions tend to invite a self-description that is feasible, compassionate, optimistic, and resourceful, while also acknowledging (at least implicitly) some of the challenges the client confronts.

Case Example

As an example of the tool of the self-characterization technique, consider the following sketch completed by a 27-year-old graduate student, Chris, who is bright and affable, and also stutters moderately. When offered a brief description of the method, he was immediately interested, and completed the written sketch in one sitting between weekly sessions. At the time, he was concentrating on overcoming the social limitations that are often associated with this stuttering, so that this form of reflective writing seemed to nicely complement the "field work" he was doing to experiment with his speaking behavior in the social world.

Chris C. has no idea what's going on. He is an individual in flux. His life used to be one of rigidity and certainty. Exposure to new thoughts, ideas, and minds has led him on a quest to let go of all the past certainties he had been holding onto with all his might. He constantly questions not only who but also what he is. He has come to realize that all of his beliefs, values, and morals have been socially constructed; in fact his whole idea of self seems to be a social construction. This makes him uncomfortable but not for the reasons one might think. It makes him uncomfortable that even though he recognizes his morals as nothing more than a social construction, he cannot violate them. He does not believe that an act can be good or evil, yet he cannot bring himself to kill, steal, cheat, or lie; he is a prisoner of his own socially constructed reality. He tries to bring this up with his friends, but they think he is crazy: "You don't want to cheat on your girlfriend or kill your brother; you sound completely healthy to me!"

Although he does not recognize an absolute self, absolute morals, or a purpose to life, this has not led to a downward spiral into complete nihilism. He recognizes that there is a middle way. He sees himself as part of the great chain of cause and effect that is nature. His choices (he would question whether he can even make choices) will become a permanent part of this chain. In this way his life is not meaningless; his actions have real consequences. One consequence does not have more intrinsic value than another. It seems to him that the only way to choose between two consequences is to make the choice that most leads to his flourishing. If his conception of flourishing is determined by society, so be it; it is the only option that he has. He sees this as the essence of choice. No one chooses suffering over flourishing. People's choices represent their best attempt to flourish. In this way he sees freewill as somewhat of an abstraction. One indeed influences one's choices, just like the shape of a cylinder will influence how it rolls down a hill. However, just as the cylinder did not determine its roundness, one's characteristics are the product of the cause and effect chain that they are a part of.

It just so happens that the suffering of others causes him to suffer. Seeing others flourish leads to his own flourishing. This is the essence of his morality. It gives his life meaning while at the same time it limits his agency and actions. He holds this contradiction within him everywhere he goes. One would think this would lead to an inner life of constant turmoil but it does not. Much like a prisoner with Stockholm syndrome, he has embraced his captor. Living according to his imposed morals makes him happy. He has let go of the need to make sense of this paradox; nothing makes sense to him anyway. When he meditates, this contradiction melts away. He recognizes that he is not a being but a process, just a part of greater nature.

Speaking of nature, Chris's reverence for nature is almost pious. He laughs as individuals busy themselves with trying to exert control over nature. Nature moves continents, creates worlds; he believes one's best bet for happiness is align one's will with that of nature. As nature has brought him into existence and endowed him with a set of morals that values limiting the suffering of others and encouraging their flourishing, he feels it is wise to embrace these values. In fact, he does not think he has any other "choice."

Despite not having any idea what is going on, Chris spends the majority of his life at peace. His day-to-day life has its ups and downs just like everyone else's but for the most part he is happy. He looks forward to his future. He tries, very hard, to be mindful of the present but does not always succeed. Deep down he is a dreamer, always thinking about other things and other times. There are certain people who are able to ground him in the present. For them he is very grateful. These are the people he calls friends and family. He loves his work, he loves the beauty of nature, but it is these individuals that make his life truly worth living.

Like most people who respond to the invitation to complete a self-characterization, Chris writes one that spans one or two pages—short enough to not be daunting, but substantial enough to offer insights into who he is and how he approaches life. Simply asking a client to read the sketch aloud or, with permission, doing so in the client's presence, can introduce a lively mutual discussion, guided by the clinician's curious questions (e.g., "How did you approach writing this? Did you plan it carefully beforehand, or undertake it in a more spontaneous way?" "Did anything in what you wrote surprise you? What if anything in the sketch would surprise others if they knew about it?" "If you could change anything about this character, what would it be? And what would you resist changing if others pressed you to do so?"). In other words, simple interest in the process of the writing and its personal meanings for the client can reveal volumes about the client's preferred style for approaching tasks (including those involved in self-change), about his or her self-understanding or capacity for insight, and about possible readiness for change and sources of resistance. In Chris's case, the picture that emerged was one that emphasized adventurousness, a capacity to "sit with" the paradoxes of the human condition, including his own, and a willingness to embrace change, as long as it was consonant with his core values. A speech therapist working alongside him might therefore collaborate in constructing homework that would prompt him to improvise in social situations, meditate, or write reflectively about the outcomes of these experiments, and follow Chris's lead in identifying tasks and assignments that would promote his own "flourishing" and that of others.

Although this alone could easily justify suggesting the self-characterization as a part of one's clinical assessment or intervention, there are also a number of "clinical guidelines"[1] for teasing still more from the sketch, which can offer optional suggestions for enhancing its value (Table 20–2). Most of these presume the clinician's willingness to do his or her own "homework," in the sense of spending half an hour or so combing through the sketch and noting

---

[1] More detailed consideration of the self-characterization as a tool for assessment and therapy can be found in the original work of Kelly (1955) as well as in the more recent work in personal construct theory (Neimeyer, 1993, 2009).

Table 20–2. Optional Guidelines for the Analysis of a Self Characterization

1. **Start with a credulous approach.** That is, don't start looking for a client's defense mechanisms, hidden weaknesses, cognitive distortions, or secret conflicts. Instead, simply try to answer the question, "What does the world look like through this person's eyes?"

2. **Observe organization.** Assume that the opening "topic sentence" of each paragraph has the greatest generality.

3. **Look for repeated terms with similar content.** These may signal key themes that are worth discussing in counseling to explore their relevance to self-change.

4. **Restate the essential themes in your own words.** This can help the clinician to grasp their basic meaning, and build a bridge of greater understanding.

5. **Assume that the writer is working at the "growing edge" of his or her self-understanding.** The areas the person chooses to discuss are usually those that contain enough uncertainty to make exploration interesting, and enough structure to make it meaningful.

6. **Examine the client's explanatory style.** How does she or he explain "what happens" in life? Are changes the consequence of personal choice and effort, are people shaped by external factors or events, or some interesting combination of these explanations?

7. **Who in the client's life supports his or her efforts? Who opposes them?** This can give the clinician an idea of who might make a good therapeutic ally, perhaps someone who could, with the client's permission, also be invited into selected sessions.

relevant patterns, which might then inform later interactions or interventions with the client. None of these guidelines is considered essential, however; rather, each is simply an optional way of "reading between the lines" of the sketch to grasp more of what clients are saying about themselves, in a way that can enhance the content and direction of their therapy.

To illustrate the use of some of these guidelines, let's imagine applying them to Chris's character sketch reproduced above. Again, each guideline is optional, and the clinician can be guided by his or her own interest as much as by the guidelines themselves.

Start with a Credulous Approach

The world to Chris looks like a bit of a mystery, but one that is more intriguing than threatening. He positions himself as a keen observer of people and events, including himself, suggesting an attitude of curiosity and humility that could serve him well in speech therapy and counseling.

Observe Organization

Read in sequence, the opening sentences of each paragraph of Chris's sketch underscore how he views the world as a complex place, but nonetheless maintains a characteristic position of engagement and interest rather than lapsing into helplessness and despair. Instead, he grounds himself in compassion and empathy for others as well as in his reverence for nature, and despite life's vicissitudes, is able to find a sense of equanimity and peace. All of these characteristics and values could provide obvious supports for efforts at self-change, suggesting an exploratory approach to therapeutic assignments, a hardiness when they do not go as well as hoped, and ways of "recharging his batteries" when they run low.

Look for Repeated Terms with Similar Content

Several clusters of related terms stand out in Chris's sketch. On the one hand, the world is presented as in *flux*, as a *process* that is constantly changing, just as the self is driven by *questions* and *new thoughts, ideas,* and *minds*. On the other hand, there is a certain stability in Chris's inner world of *beliefs, values,* and *morals*, which confer a *middle way* sort of *purpose*—to advance his mutual *flourishing* with others and in this way relieve their *suffering* and perhaps his own *inner turmoil*. *Mindfulness* and contact with *nature*, of which he is a part, are invoked as important routes to *peace* in the midst of *paradox*. Efforts at change should therefore respect these core values and purposes, as well as draw on the resources provided by his meditation to help him not take himself too seriously when he encounters occasional setbacks.

Examine the Client's Explanatory Style

Chris implies a complex and seemingly paradoxical philosophy to explain the events and actions of his life, on the one hand situating them within timeless ideologies of "the great chain of cause and effect" as well as a contemporary consideration of one's own life and identity as a "social construction." On the other hand, he readily acknowledges the sense of personal agency and choice with which he implements his values in concrete situations. Both of these features—the recognition that our life stories are "coauthored" by larger forces beyond our control, but that we also have a hand in how they turn out—could be useful in helping him sort through the inevitable vagaries of attempts at fostering fluency or self confidence, even in the presence of suffering.

Who in the Client's Life Supports His or Her Efforts? Who Opposes Them?

Though they are unnamed, it is clear that Chris's family and friends are a great source of support and meaning for which he is genuinely grateful. Thus, engaging them in therapy and counseling (perhaps in practicing newly acquired skills, accompanying him into new situations, or alternatively standing back and allowing him to engage such situations on his own) could represent a logical extension of his individual treatment.

Concluding Thoughts

In summary, the self-characterization represents a straightforward but surprisingly rich tool for looking more deeply into the story that clients tell themselves and others about who they are, what they value, and how they cope. Whether used systematically or impressionistically in therapy with adults with communication disorders, self-characterization can be a source of considerable insight for client and therapist alike, and can help in co-constructing an approach to treatment that respects and uses the unique resources that clients bring to the process of change.

Frequently Asked Questions

Q: If a client cannot write—either because of physical limitations or literacy deficits—can the self-characterization be elicited verbally, recorded, and then transcribed?

A: Very often. For example, with a 9-year-old client, a clinician might take dictation in session, prompting occasionally with additional questions (e.g., "What else does Jasmine like to do? Who does she choose as friends, and why? Is there anything that makes her feel bad at times?"). With adolescents and adults, electronic dictation software that is widely available on smart phones, tablets, and computers can serve a similar purpose without additional clinician prompting. Having a written rather than simply an oral transcription of the recording is an advantage in promoting the "self-distancing" mentioned earlier in this chapter, as well as possibly setting the stage for *fixed role therapy*, discussed in Chapter 21. It can also assist the clinician in reviewing the content and structure of the sketch more fully, as illustrated in this chapter.

Q: Can the self-characterization process be used in a situation where caregivers write about the person under their care (e.g., a parent writing about a child with autism; a spouse writing about her husband who is now nonverbal following a stroke)?

A: Certainly, as long as the clinician keeps in mind that the constructs in the sketch are those of the writer and not the client! Still, this can be very revealing and helpful in a family consultation context: How does the caregiver view the person in their care? For example, if a mother is writing about her young son with autism, does she depict him as *fascinated with the physical world, focused, disciplined* and *independent*, or as *demanding, impossible to understand, socially awkward* and *rigid*? In the latter case, counseling might well concentrate on the mother's narrative about her child, as well as on communication training for the boy himself. Davis and her colleagues (Davis, Stroud, & Green, 1989) suggest that in such an application of this method that caregivers simply be asked "to describe the personality or behavior" of their family member as fully as possible, as they "know [the loved one] better than anyone." They then offer guidelines similar to those in Table 20-2, but with the added suggestion that the clinician take special note of any words that describe how writers feel about the child or family member in their care.

References

Davis, H., Stroud, A., & Green, L. (1989). Child characterization sketch. *International Journal of Personal Construct Psychology, 2*, 323–337.

Kelly, G. A. (1955). *The psychology of personal constructs*. New York, NY: Norton.

Kross, E., & Ayduk, O. (2010). Making meaning out of negative experiences by self-distancing. *Current Directions in Psychological Science, 20*, 187–191. doi: 10.1177/0963721411408883

Neimeyer, R. A. (1993). Constructivist approaches to the measurement of meaning. In G. J. Neimeyer (Ed.), *Constructivist assessment: A casebook* (pp. 58–103). Newbury Park: CA: Sage.

Neimeyer, R. A. (2009). *Constructivist psychotherapy*. London, UK & New York, NY: Routledge.

21

EXPERIMENTING
WITH EXPERIENCE

*Chris Constantino, Robert A.
Neimeyer, and Anthony DiLollo*

Clients for Whom the Tool Is Appropriate

In this chapter we discuss therapy techniques that experiment with client's roles and behaviors. This type of work is appropriate for any chronic communication disorder. Individuals who have been living with long-term developmental disorders, such as childhood apraxia of speech, developmental stuttering, congenital hearing loss, and craniofacial anomalies, as well as individuals with acquired disorders, such as acquired apraxia of speech, dysarthria, aphasia, dysphonia, acquired hearing loss, and cognitive-communication disorders can benefit from playfully perturbing their everyday roles and behaviors. These techniques occur over a time frame of several weeks and would, therefore, only be applicable to clients who see the same clinician regularly.

Materials Needed

These techniques require both the clinician and client to have an open mind and a willingness to engage in playful, experiential therapy methods. Experimenting with experience requires active participation in novel identities and behaviors over a fixed time period outside of therapy; consequently the most important resource for these methods is time. For some tools such as fixed-role therapy, a prior character sketch (see Chapter 20) is required as a basis for the new role, whereas for others a simple method of charting behaviors can be helpful, as illustrated below.

In some capacity or another, all of our clients come to us seeking change. If they were content with the way their lives were going, they would not bother to seek professional assistance. Narrative constructivist psychology offers insight into this process of change and gives advice for how clinicians can join with clients to accomplish it. Counseling is understood as an intervention in meaning-making and in giving voice to new narratives. New constructs can be formed and poles realigned all within the backdrop of an emancipated life story—one free from domination by the problem (see Chapter 5 for a description of the bipolar nature of constructs).

Constructivist counselors see the process of change as experiential rather than intellectual. According to constructive alternativism, as outlined in Chapter 5, meaning is changed when an individual experiments with a different way of being in the world. This playful experimentation challenges an individual's current construct system, resulting in growth and modification of existing constructs. In real concrete ways, it shows our clients that alternative ways of living are available to them.

Experimentation can be encouraged in a number of ways and different capacities. Clients can adopt a whole new role or an imaginary identity for a fixed amount of time, a procedure known as *fixed-role therapy* (Kelly, 1955/1991; Neimeyer et al., 2003). This global approach to experimentation can lead to insightful change and a rapid sense of empowerment and agency. However, overall role enactment is not always possible and, even when it is, clients sometimes need extra help to change specific behaviors. For these cases, clients can employ more targeted experimentation with certain behaviors that are of interest, but with the same playful, experimental attitude. Regardless of whether we are experimenting with roles or with specific behaviors, such exploratory therapy can be both fun and exciting. Our clients are encouraged to actually go out and be the personal scientists that Kelly (1955/1991) originally envisioned them to be; they are *experimenting with experience.*

Fixed-Role Therapy: Experimenting with Identity

Roles are not a foreign concept to the literature of communication sciences and disorders. Sheehan (1970) famously saw stuttering as a disorder characterized primarily by role conflict. People who stutter were described as trying to live the role of a fluent speaker. In an effort to fulfill this role, they attempt to minimize their stuttering through avoidance and secondary behaviors. The unfortunate result of this is increased tension, more frequent stuttering, and a greatly restricted lifestyle.

Fixed-role therapy[1] can be used to encourage experimentation with different ways of being. It is a playful method of enacting and performing alternative identities. This is always done for a fixed period of time determined prior to the enactment. Because there is a set time limit, the clients have the added relief of knowing that they are not making permanent changes. They do not have to actually become someone else, but only pretend to be for a short time, like someone going to a costume party or taking part in a play or skit. Knowing they will not have to wear their new role for very long makes it easier for them to don the new identity and see how it feels. Importantly, in this constructivist version of role-play, the idea is not to "correct" some faulty cognitions on the part of the client or to practice new behavioral skills, as in most forms of cognitive behavioral therapy (CBT). Instead, the goal is "serious play," simply experiencing the world of communication differently for a time, to convey how even one's sense of oneself as a social

---

[1] For a detailed discussion of fixed-role therapy, readers are referred to Chapter 8, Volume 1 of Kelly's original work (1955) and the more recent work by Robert A Neimeyer et al. (2003).

being could be approached differently in the future. This "make believe" framework often lets people approach change with less threat, knowing they can always revert to more familiar ways of being when the experiment is over.

Fixed-role therapy requires the development of an enactment sketch. Enactment sketches are gentle and playful invitations for clients to adopt a new role, a script for the client's future performance. Enactment sketches are often developed from self-characterizations (see Chapter 20). It can be fruitful to have the client write a self-characterization before the clinician attempts to write an enactment sketch because this provides a gauge of the client's willingness to experiment with new viewpoints and attitudes. Such sketches also give clinicians a good idea of how the client is currently viewing and doing life, so that they can design an alternative identity that is distinct from the old one without contradicting it, or depicting an overly idealized alternative. A thorough discussion of this process can be found elsewhere (Neimeyer & Winter, 2006).

The sketch that the clinician comes up with should represent an individual who confronts similar (though not identical) challenges as the client but tackles them from a different perspective. These new perspectives should be mindful of the client's core constructs and should not attempt to perturb them too much; that is, the new sketch should respect the client's core values. Instead, peripheral constructs can be altered and rearranged. In this way the new role can be thought of as "orthogonal" to the old role, in other words, it is neither entirely familiar nor entirely foreign (Neimeyer & Winter, 2006). The client must be consulted during this development process. Only the client can judge whether seemingly minor tweaks to his or her self-characterization are too big, too small, or as like Goldilocks said when checking out the beds of the three bears, "just right." In addition, the enactment sketch should paint the picture of a well-rounded individual, complete with quirks and eccentricities as well as strengths.

It is important that the enactment sketch be supported with concrete examples of behavior for the client to perform. These can be in the form of explicit instructions about how the new character

Table 21–1. Hypothetical Fixed-Role Characters and Their Prominent Characteristics

Name	Role description
Andy Vidual	One-of-a-kind, self-enhancing personality
Anna Graham	An intriguing puzzle to others
Anna Lytic	Intellectually intense; always looking for a deeper meaning
Bobbie Sox	Fun-loving and unpretentious
Freida Choose	Constructs many alternatives for action
Greg Garious	Mr. Sociability; life-of-the-party
Ira Knee	Witty, with a knack for seeing the absurd side of things
Jerry Atric	Copes resiliently with losses of aging
Mike Quest	A man with a mission
Otto Kinetic	Always on the move
Phil Anthropic	Generous to a fault; loves all mankind
Polly Gonn	Many-sided personality
Reed Define	Likes reframing situations in novel ways
Sally Forth	Oriented to an adventurous future
Sharon Sharalike	Seeks "give and take" in close relationships
Taylor Made	Fits into his niche in life perfectly
Wanda A. Round	Undirected but happy-go-lucky

interacts with other people, what kinds of places he or she frequents, and what his or her hobbies are. The more specific these instructions are, the easier it will be for the client to adopt the role, for example by suggesting particular books, movies, or restaurants the new character enjoys. The character described in the enactment sketch can also be given a name to make him or her more real; perhaps a name can be even be playfully created to suggest some key character traits to make the role more memorable (Table 21-1). Try to create a character that the client would actually be interested in getting to know better. The client should feel like he or she is really trying to step into this other person's shoes for a fixed period of time, usually a couple of weeks, during which the counselor meets with the client to help him or her practice the new role by enacting the part of others in his or her life while the client adopts the new character. Importantly, the enactment sketch need not even directly address the communication disorder, but can instead work with new communication patterns by implication, as by prescribing social behaviors (e.g., being inquisitive about the outlooks of others, or enjoying the sharing of a good joke) that would naturally lead the client to communicate differently. This indirect approach can be especially helpful if a client is making some progress with the technical aspects of treatment, so expanding his or her identity in a direction that implies greater communicative competence could help consolidate these germinal changes.

There are other ways to develop enactment sketches, including some that more directly implicate changes in communication patterns. Perhaps one of the most useful methods is to have clients imagine themselves as they would be without their communication disorders (Winter, 1992). If they have an acquired disorder (e.g., aphasia, hearing loss) they can be prompted to remember what things were like before the disorder. If they have a developmental disorder (e.g., developmental stuttering, childhood apraxia of speech) they can be asked to imagine what things would be like if they lost their symptoms or had never had them in the first place. They also can be prompted to imagine what they would be like if therapy could be completely successful at treating their disorder. An example of this technique is given below.

Case Example

Brad is a 55-year-old man who has recently been diagnosed with adductor spasmodic dysphonia. He receives occasional injections of botulinum toxin (Botox) which manage some of his symptoms but he still speaks with a noticeably strained, strangled vocal quality. Brad is a high level manager at the company he works for. Before his voice disorder, he really enjoyed his job. He was seen as a "tough love" kind of boss, one his workers respected, for pushing them hard while maintaining a good relationship. Since developing his voice disorder, he feels he has lost control of his job. He resorts to e-mail instead of face-to-face meetings and suspects he is losing the esteem of his workers. He worries about his ability to perform his job with the same success that he enjoyed in the past. He is a practicing Catholic and used to take an active role in singing at his church. While singing, his vocal quality improves but his dysphonia and the Botox injections have drastically decreased his vocal range. As a result, he can no longer sing in his church choir without feeling embarrassed. This greatly upsets Brad as singing was a large part of his identity. He often described singing and worship as his two favorite activities. He wishes there were a way he could be still be involved in his church, but singing seems to be out of the question. In general, Brad feels as though he is retreating into himself. He spends less time socializing and more time at home with his two chocolate Labradors. Ever since he was a little boy, he has enjoyed building model cars and trains. To this day he is an avid model builder and his hobby has now become his main source of enjoyment in life. He loves going home after work and working on his current model. Table 21–2 shows an enactment sketch for "Lou K. Shush" that Brad and his clinician came up with together.

Brad adopted the role of Lou for two weeks. He was instructed to read the sketch each morning upon waking up and each night before sleep. He was also asked to journal about his experiences as Lou. During this time Lou and his clinician had two sessions each week where they meet to discuss his experiences. On the last day Lou wrote a letter of advice to Brad wishing him the best of luck in therapy. The next therapy session Brad was himself again. The clinician read his letter out loud to him and they discussed what Brad had learned from Lou. Brad's experience as Lou opened up options for him to live life more like the way he wanted to live. Although he hated karaoke, he found Toastmasters a valuable experience and was appreciative of his renewed involvement in his

Table 21–2. "Lou K. Shush" Engagement Sketch

Lou K. Shush has an energetic outlook on life. He lives by the maxim, *work hard, play hard*. During the work week, he works diligently trying to manage the people in his company. The excessive demands and fast-paced nature of his job mean he often cannot wait for his coworkers to return e-mails; instead he often calls their office phones directly. Some of his coworkers find his style of communication confrontational, but he knows it is necessary. On weeknights Lou likes to relax and spend time with his two dogs. He takes them for walks in Rochedale Park, near his house. This is usually time spent alone with himself and his two companions, but every once in a while he crosses paths with another park-goer. When this happens, Lou is happy to introduce himself and talk about how beautiful the park looks at night or whatever else comes up. He loves conversations with strangers.

During weekends, Lou K. Shush tries to stay busy. He is an active Toastmaster and takes pride in his ability to keep audiences on the edge of their seats, despite his voice disorder. Friday nights he goes to Murphy's, his favorite bar, with a few of his friends. Friday at Murphy's is karaoke night. With some prodding, his friends can usually get him to sing. He pretends he doesn't like the attention he gets from his singing but he really does. On Saturdays and Sundays, he typically rests and spends time on his model-building hobby. Lou is an active member of his church and often volunteers to give the readings Sunday mornings.

church—a "bonus" from his experiment in being gregarious that was not explicitly emphasized in his sketch.

The Power of Paradox: Experimenting with Problem Behaviors

Sometimes clients may find focusing on particular behaviors beneficial. This can be done as part of a broader fixed-role enactment or as a targeted therapy where there is only a single behavior of interest. Typically behaviors that require targeted attention have become habitual and automatic over time or are behaviors that the client is really struggling to alter. These behaviors may have become intimately entwined with the clients' sense of self and not amenable to indirect experimentation.

Our clients are aware of the stigma that comes with being labeled disabled by society. Disability is regularly conceptualized as a detraction from the ideal human state (Campbell, 2001). People with disabilities are seen as less than ideal or less than optimal. Not surprisingly, people with communication disorder will frequently go through a great deal of effort to pass as a non-disabled individual, though ironically this can lead to global restrictions in lifestyle and quality of life. For this reason, the specific behaviors we often want our clients to perform involve purposely embracing their role as a person with a disability. Two examples are presented below.

Voluntary Stuttering

Developmental stuttering is a disorder that manifests itself in involuntary disruptions to the forward flow of an individual's speech. A real stutter is an event that causes speakers to lose control of their speech mechanism while speaking. This experience in and of itself can be jarring to the speaker as it can often be unexpected; however, what is perhaps even more jarring is that the speaker does not always know when he will regain control. In other words, he does not know how long the stutter will last. This is quite a detriment to speaking. The combined fear of losing control and not being able to regain it causes many individuals who stutter to speak with a great deal of fear and tension. This manner of speaking inevitably leads to increased stuttering, contributing to a vicious circle. In addition, many people who stutter develop an extensive repertoire of avoidance behaviors to try to hide their stuttering from their listeners, which can also lead to more stuttering. This combination of behaviors can result in a very complicated speaking pattern. Voluntary stuttering, a technique developed at the University of Iowa by Bryng Bryngelson and made popular by Wendell Johnson and Charles Van Riper (Bloodstein, 1995; Bryngelson, 1934), can be used to address both of the issues mentioned above. Voluntary stuttering occurs when a person who stutters "stutters" on purpose. Of course, it cannot be a real stutter as a real stutter is involuntary, and for this reason the technique is sometimes called pseudostuttering. By using voluntary stuttering, the speaker is able to experience stuttering without the loss of control. She can begin to experiment with different ways to stutter, ways that are easier and less tense. Voluntary stuttering also contradicts avoidance mechanisms. Purposely displaying a behavior is the antithesis of hiding it, returning a measure of choice and control by paradoxically embracing and inviting the problem.

Voluntary Miscomprehension

People with hearing impairments deal not only with discrimination surrounding disability but also frequently with discrimination surrounding age. It is often seen as the responsibility of the individual to get amplification if he or she has a hearing loss. Many people with hearing loss have internalized this sentiment, frequently apologizing for not hearing what some else has said. Clients are trapped in a no-win situation: a person with a hearing impairment who does not seek amplification is blamed for the communication breakdown; yet an individual with visible hearing aids is stigmatized as old and disabled.

For this reason individuals with hearing loss, with and without amplification, will often fake comprehension during conversation (Wallhagen, 2010). This leads to further communication breakdowns and a diminished quality of life. It is important that people with hearing loss be comfortable revealing that there has been a failure in communication, regardless of whether or not they choose to seek amplification. Asking a communication partner to repeat something is hard. It can instantly make the individual vulnerable to stigma. There is also no guarantee that the individual will comprehend the message when it is repeated the second time, or third, or fourth. The inability to comprehend a message can be an embarrassing and shameful experience for people with hearing loss.

Clients with hearing loss can be invited to pretend that they did not understand a speaking partner when they did in fact understand the message. This puts the communication breakdown directly in the hands of the client. Much like voluntary stuttering, pretending not to understand a message allows clients to be in control of a situation in which they typically have no control. This makes the exercise less stressful than asking for clarification when they did not understand the message. There is no risk of not understanding it the second time. Clients can ask for clarification on their own terms. This allows them to get comfortable with different ways of asking and also desensitizes them to the behavior.

Motivation

The trouble with each of these suggestions is that each asks clients to do the thing that they fear the most. This can be downright terrifying. For persons who are attending therapy to help minimize the impact of a hearing loss or stuttering on their lives, the last thing they want to hear is that they should purposely display their symptoms. In order to make the exercise less intimating, we recommend framing it as a game or performance—very much in the spirit of fixed-role therapy. For example, clients and clinicians can practice the behavior together, with each member playing both parts, before suggesting that the client try the voluntary behavior spontaneously with the clinic receptionist or another staff member before heading out into the "real world." Having the clinician voluntarily speak disfluently or feign difficulty hearing the client can help "level the playing field" and destigmatize the behavior, while also enhancing the counselor's empathy for the client's situation. Once the client is onboard with the experiment, the two can come up with playful objectives to attempt, rather than a strict counting of target behaviors. Much as with more formal fixed-role therapy, these single behavior performances should also be restricted to a fixed time. Clients will be more likely to embrace a challenging performance if it is only for a week or two, during which they should have consistent access to counseling sessions (perhaps twice a week) to offer a "secure base" for their experiments.

If the performance is kept fun and interesting, it will be much more motivating to the client. This can be done by discussing and implementing a progression system in which the individual tries to increase or generalize the behavior over time. This progress does not have to be simply performing the behavior more frequently. The client can be challenged to perform the task in a different situation each day, in different settings, at different times of the day, or in different manners. If the objectives are challenging but fun, they will encourage the client to think about how to accomplish the performance at the beginning of each day. For example, a woman with a hearing loss can implement a system in which she has to increase the number of repeated times she asks for clarification with a single individual each day for a week (asking one person to repeat what they said seven times can be quite the experiment!). Another challenge for a client with hearing loss may be to try to make a communication partner laugh with a misunderstanding of an utterance, as with one playful father who "misheard" his grade school son's remark at the dinner table referring to a friend who was a "practicing nudist" (rather than Buddhist), contributing to general hilarity in the ensuing conversation. The progression would be to try to make an additional person laugh every day for a week. Another example, from one of the authors' own experience with stuttering, follows.

Case Example

Figure 21–1 shows a week's results of a two-tiered progression system I (Chris) used for voluntary stuttering. My goal for each day was to either voluntarily stutter in more scenarios than I did on the previous day or to have more voluntary stutters in one particular scenario than I did on the previous day. Even though I did increase my overall frequency over all three days, this was not the intended goal. I chose this system because simply increasing the frequency of voluntary stuttering every day would have soon become burdensome.

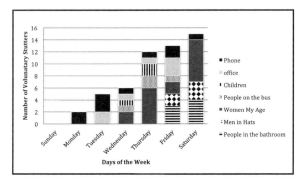

Figure 21–1. Frequency of voluntary stuttering in various scenarios.

Also, the idea of finding new and interesting scenarios in which to voluntarily stutter made the assignment more thought provoking and fun. Some days I would look for different categories of people to voluntarily stutter with, such as children, people on the bus, or people in the office. On other days I would try to stutter more times with a particular category of people with whom I had felt nervous stuttering on a previous day (e.g., a woman my age). Within a few days, I found myself coming up with amusing categories of people with whom I could try to stutter, like people in the bathroom and men with hats. When the behavior your client is trying to perform becomes entertaining and exciting, then clearly progress has been made! I concluded the week of performance feeling more relaxed, amused, and efficacious in communication situations, which probably contributed to my greater fluency at other times.

Concluding Thoughts

Constructivist counseling entails "trying on" new constructs as well as new behaviors, often while wearing the protective mask of make-believe. Cultivating a playful attitude toward time-limited experiments with clients can help lift some of the deadly seriousness with which they approach their problem, ironically magnifying its power in their attempts to avoid it. By approaching life differently for a time, and perhaps even arranging to display the very problems they fearfully avoid, clients can often develop greater flexibility, and begin to reduce the shame with which they perform the problem. The results of such experiences can make for some lively reflective conversations between clients and their counselors, and begin to win back a measure of control from the dominant narrative of disability.

Frequently Asked Questions

Q: How long should clients adopt a fixed role?
A: Typically two to three weeks is enough time for an individual to benefit from experiencing a novel identity.

Q: When holding therapy sessions while doing fixed-role therapy, should the individual keep up the performance?

A: It depends. If the client is very comfortable performing his new role, he can be invited to stay in character during therapy sessions. It could be a great learning experience for the client to experience therapy from another perspective. However, if the client is struggling with the exercise, therapy sessions can be used as a way to troubleshoot and talk about problems he is having with the performance.

Q: How long should clients experiment with specific behaviors?

A: Experimenting with specific behaviors is a more targeted exercise than experimenting with an identity. For this reason only a week or two of performance should be necessary for clients to get a feel for the exercise. If they find the behavior helpful, they should be encouraged to continue performing it. If they find the behavior very difficult, they can be given a respite after four or five days and invited to perform the behavior again in the future. However, it is usually beneficial to try out the new behavior for at least a few days until the client experiences some level of desensitization to the experience, because a quick retreat from the anxiety of trying something new can reinforce shame and associated avoidance coping.

Q: Should clients keep a written or typed record of target behaviors?

A: Yes, charting or journaling about their experiments allows clients to track their progress and motivates them to progress in the exercise. It can be easy to fall back into old habits in between therapy sessions. When clients keep a record of their progress, it also serves as a reminder of what they are trying to accomplish while not in the therapy room, and often helps them consolidate the *action iMoments* associated with the exercise into *reflection* and *reconceptualization iMoments* that help them hold onto subtle changes in their social identity in the world of communication.

References

Bloodstein, O. (1995). *A handbook on stuttering*. San Diego, CA: Singular Publishing Group.

Bryngelson, B. (1934). Voluntary stuttering. *Proceedings from: The Professional Discussions of the Ninth Annual Convention of the American Speech Correction Association, 4*, 35–38.

Campbell, F. A. (2001). Inciting legal fictions: Disability's date with ontology and the ableist body of the law. *Griffith Law Review, 10*, 42–62.

Kelly, G. A. (1955/1991). *The psychology of personal constructs*. New York, NY: Routledge.

Neimeyer, R. A., & Winter, D. A. (2006). Personal construct therapy. In N. Kazantzis & L. L'Abate (Eds.), *Handbook of homework assignments in psychotherapy*. New York, NY: Kluwer.

Sheehan, J. G. (1970). *Stuttering: Research and therapy*. New York, NY: Harper & Row.

Wallhagen, M. I. (2010). The stigma of hearing loss. *The Gerontologist, 50*(1), 66–75.

Winter, D. A. (1992). *Personal construct psychology in clinical practice: Theory, research and applications*. New York, NY: Routledge.

22

CHAIR WORK

Robert A. Neimeyer, Chris Constantino, and Anthony DiLollo

Clients for Whom the Tool Is Appropriate

Adolescents and adults with a range of expressive or hearing disorders can benefit from the clarity of performing a spoken dialogue with their problem as a basis for renegotiating their relationship to it. However, for very young children, the perspective-taking required can make chair work more daunting, and for clients with aphasia, coginitive-lingustic disorders, or other severe difficulties with oral communication, an alternative way of exploring the role of the problem in their lives could be more fruitful.

Materials Needed

Optimally the method requires three chairs, two directly facing one another and a third at right angles to them, for the counselor. All three chairs should be at a comfortable conversational distance.

Description

Although we typically think of ourselves as "individuals," implying that we are indivisible, fully coherent personalities, it is rare that we are of a "single mind" about anything! Indeed, we often catch ourselves arguing with ourselves about one course of action or another, feeling ambivalent about a given relationship, or chiding ourselves for some mistake that we have made. Even when each of us is not in internal conflict or contradiction, we typically function as a *dialogical self* (Hermans & Gieser, 2012), that is, as a being with many different "voices" capable of engaging one another in inner conversations. In fact, the ability to *externalize* problems as something separate from ourselves to which we have a relationship draws on this same idea. *Chair work*, adapted from emotion focused therapy (Greenberg, 2010), simply takes this idea one step further by suggesting that we literally grant the problem a voice, and enter into a conversation with it.

Getting Started

Viewed from a dialogical perspective, anything capable of being personified can be given voice (Rowan, 2010), and this certainly applies to our symptoms or problems. Thus, a client with a communication disorder could enter into a meaningful dialogue with his or her anxiety, deafness, stuttering, or any number of other discrete difficulties once they are externalized as something distinguishable from themselves as people. In chairing, the problem is given a place in a chair opposite the client at a comfortable conversational distance, with the therapist seated at right angles to the client so as to be out of the client's line of sight (Figure 22–1). Readiness to engage the problem in conversation can be suggested by the client's remark (e.g., "I don't know why I can't get over the anxiety"), to which the clinician might respond with an invitation to a dialogue with the symptom (e.g., "Hmm. I have a crazy idea. What if we were to ask Anxiety that very question [gesturing to the empty chair]: 'Why can't I get over you?' What more would you like to

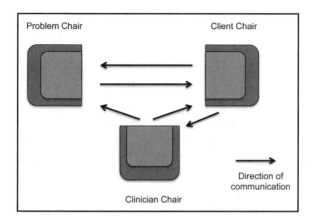

Figure 22–1. Typical configuration for chair work.

say to Anxiety about that?"). If the client has already grown familiar with externalizing conversations, the step to performance of the dialogue is typically an easy one.

In the process of introducing this method to a client who is less familiar with it, a simple orientation can be provided in a couple of sentences. For example, the clinician might say, "If Anxiety were sitting over here in this chair (gesturing), listening into our conversation, what would you tell him about how you feel about his presence in your life? How does it feel to have Anxiety intrude into so many of your conversations with people?" The clinician would then look to the empty chair, in effect directing the client's eyes in the same direction, and avoiding the implicit demand for the client to maintain eye contact with him or her. If the client begins, "I'd guess I'd tell him that . . ." the clinician would gently interrupt and prompt, "Try saying that directly to him. 'What I want to tell you is. . . .'" The counselor then listens, prompting occasionally, in order to help the client share a full and honest statement of his or her feeling or questions. For example, if the client says, "You just make me uncomfortable all the time," the counselor might prompt, "Tell him more about how he makes you feel." Usually, within a minute or two, the client is delving honestly into previously unexpressed emotions about, questions for, or protests against the problem, in a way that clearly invites a "response" from the problem being addressed.

Giving Voice to the Problem

To facilitate a two-way exchange, the clinician simply gestures toward the empty chair, saying something like, "Why don't you come over here now," and as the client does so, adding, ". . . and loan the Anxiety your own voice. What would Anxiety say back to this person who says, 'You make me so uncomfortable in my own skin! I'm tired of living in fear of you! Why can't you just leave me alone?'" (quoting a few poignant phrases from the client's statement). The clinician then looks to the client's now empty chair, implicitly inviting Anxiety to do the talking. Again prompted toward directness and honesty by the counselor, Anxiety might say something like, "The truth is, you need me around. I'm the one who tells you when a social situation isn't safe. And I'll never leave you like others will." Listening for a natural pause that would call for a response, the clinician would then direct the client back to his or her own seat to respond: "What would you say to Anxiety about that, that you need him, and he'll always stay with you?" The conversation then continues in this way until the client has gone back and forth two or three times, until reaching a kind of insight about the role of the problem in his or her life, or until the client has renegotiated in some useful way his or her relation to the problem. In the context of communication disorders, this usually occurs within 10 to 15 minutes.

Processing the Chair Work

When the clinician senses that chairing has yielded some important material that deserves further reflection, often signaled by the client's glancing back to him or her as if to invite such discussion, the counselor can "un-stage" the chair work by directing the client back to his or her own seat and saying, "Why don't we take a few minutes to discuss what just unfolded here? As you found yourself going back and forth between these two positions, what caught your attention? What observations do you have about your conversation with Anxiety?" Often the resulting insights are surprising: "I never realized what a bully he was!" or "He's right, I do need him, he does protect me in a way. But I'm not a child any more, and I don't need him to make me so afraid! If he'd just clue me in to when a situation could be difficult, I can find a way to handle it." Engaging in another 5 or 10 minutes of conversation about the chair work, clinician and client are then in a good position to see what the "next step" in renegotiating the relationship with the problem might be, perhaps encouraging the client to write a Dear John letter to Anxiety (Chapter 18), practice mindfulness (Chapter 25), listen to the voice of Anxiety with less reactivity, or simply plan a "check in" with Anxiety the next week in another chair work conversation, the way couples therapists invite partners to remain engaged with one another constructively until each understands the other and they reach a resolution. Whether used to support externalization, provide a context for generating iMoments (especially of a reflective and protest type), or to process with the problem novel outcomes generated by other technical or adaptive interventions, chairing can be a flexible and creative way of fostering clarity and change.

Case Example

Chris is a 28-year-old man with moderate developmental stuttering who has participated in technical therapies and self-therapy to modify his speech for much of his life. Recently he has been concentrating on adaptive dimensions of the condition, greatly reducing secondary anxiety and negative self-evaluation associated with its emergence in social conditions. His changing relationship with stuttering suggested the utility of using chair work to foster a direct conversation with the externalized condition in the course of a session with the counselor (Bob). Their beginning position for the chair work matches that depicted in Figure 22-1.

Bob: Hey, Chris. It's good to see you again this week.

Chris: Good to see you too, Bob.

Bob: Yeah . . . so I found myself curious after our last session about how your relationship with stuttering has been progressing.

Chris: I've been d__doing a-a lot of thinking about um aaa-about my stuttering and about how I've been tri-tri-treating it, uh, over these years. And I used to really look at . . . look at my stuttering as something that was, something that I had to *fight* against. [Bob: mmhmm] Something that I had to overcome, um, and thth-this past w-week I've really been rr-*rethinking* [Bob: ahh] th-that relationship.

Bob: So not so much a *combative* relationship of fighting against it but somehow just, seeing it differently? In different terms?

Chris: Yeah, I almost feel like I've been *mistreating* it in a way.

Bob: Mistreating your stuttering?

Chris: Yeah, I've been treating it as something that had to be . . . had to be hidden. That was sss-inherently *negative*. [Bob: ahh] Um, and it was almost like . . . it was like this *pariah* that I had to get ___*out* of my life and it's no wonder that uhhh, it is no wonder that my stuttering rerrerr-*rebelled* against that.

Bob: Ahhh, yeah, sure, because no one would want to be just put out in the cold in that way, just like a, a *scapegoat* almost. [Chris: yeah] Just, uh, chased out. So, with this, it almost sounds like an *apology* is in order!

Chris: I feel like that. Yes!

Getting Started

In the opening minutes of the session, Chris's significant "rethinking" of his relationship with his speech pattern, combined with his rich personification of Stuttering (as a "pariah" who is "rebelling" against Chris's "mistreatment" of him) alerts Bob to the relevance of chair work to sort out the history of the relationship, which appears to be on the threshold of reconstruction. He then simply does an *acceptance check* to assess Chris's readiness to undertake this work, without an elaborate psycho-educational preface that would merely increase his anxiety.

> **Bob:** Uh huh. Well you know, I, we've been talking a little bit about this idea of externalizing the problem. And, of course, the terms that you've been speaking in here, where you've really conjured an almost living relationship with the stuttering, a relationship that is undergoing review and revision, um, just suggests to me that we might take one step further in that direction and invite you to have a conversation *with the stuttering*. Would that be of interest to you?
>
> **Chris:** Yyyyyy-yeah I th_ I think that'd be interesting.
>
> **Bob:** Well, why don't we give that a try if you feel ready for that. [Chris: Okay.] And my idea is a simple one, that we place the stuttering in this chair [gesturing to empty chair across from Chris], in this *comfortable* chair (smile and laughter from Chris), alright [Chris: mmhmm], and that we have a chance maybe first for you to say something about the results of your rethinking of this relationship. About the, you know, the struggle to fight against the, the stuttering, to fight against it or him. Would it have a gender, by the way?
>
> **Chris:** (sighs and clears throat in thought) I guess because I've been so intent on _trying to negate it, I haven't even given any, given any thought ttt-to what it would be like personified [Bob: uh huh], um, but I'm inclined to give it a _m-male gender just___for congruency with my own gender.
>
> **Bob:** Ok. So, let's begin maybe with an invitation for you to say something to him about how you've been treating him and how about how you're thinking of treating him differently now.
>
> **Chris:** Alright.
>
> **Bob:** What would you, how would you begin that conversation with Stuttering?

Chris: Hello, Stuttering. I-I know that ww-we've had our battles over the years and um we haven't always gotten aaa-along. We could even say we have never really gotten along. Um . . . and I used to think that was entirely your fault [Bob: mmm], and that yy-you were controlling, controlling my life, and taking hold of my throat and not letting me sss-speak. [Bob: Yeah.] But now I realize that, um, it's not that simple, and that the way I treated you didn't give you much of a *choice* in how to respond ti-ti-ti-to me. [Bob. Mmm] So . . .

Here Chris falls silent for a moment, seemingly unsure of how to proceed. To help him, Bob simply asks him to repeat the last significant bit of his statement, which seemed to acknowledge his own role in configuring a negative relationship with Stuttering.

Bob: Say that to him again, "I realized I didn't give you much of a *choice* as to how to respond to me."

Chris: Do you want me to repeat it in the same way?

Bob: Yeah, or just in a way that is natural for you. Maybe you would add to that or change something about that.

Chris: Okay . . . I, ____just like any other part of w-who I am, you have certain charac__characteristics and ss-certain needs that uh need to manifest, and I tried to *push you down*, tried to *hide* you, tried to *not let you ssss-see the light of day*. And . . . it's no wonder that, um . . . you wouldn't let me speak; because that's all you could have done under those ss-circumstances. [Bob: mmm] And if we had worked together instead of trying to, trying to *fight* each other, I think we could have had a much better relationship.

Bob: I wonder if you could just say that piece again, "I want to find a way of working *with* you, not *against* you."

Chris: I wanna find a way of working *with* you and not *against* you. I want us to, I want to . . . whenever I would think about you being part of me, it was always um, *temporary*, it was always something I hoped __would go away and I never really fully *integrated* you into my sense of self. Anytime I accomplished anything it was always in__, it was always in sss-sss-sss-spite of you aa-and it was never, it was never ww-*we* who accomplished it, ii-it was always *me*. [Bob: mm] Um (clears throat), and I feel like that was a *mistake* and you've *taught me a lot* ov-ov-ov-over the years and to not give you credit fff-for that is misleading.

Bob: Tell him more about what he's taught you over these years as you reflect on it.

Chris: I immediately think to just, what I value in my life. Um, you . . . you forced me to not_care about what other people thought about me, cause i-if I did I would have gone kk-criiii-crazy. Um, you taught me about how to figure out what was really *important* in my life and to set my p-priorities to try to accomplish, try to accomplish those goals insss_sstead of caring about mmmm-my reputation and accomplishing other people's goals that would increase my reputation. Um, you've also caused me a lot of *pain*, and I think I've grown from that pain and now situations that um might be, could be hard in the future, I think I'm better prepared to handle because of you. [Bob: mm] And you've also just taught me to *accept things* as th___ as they are and not hope for things to be other than they can possibly be. Um, I've always_wanted to be__be__be me *without* you, but you've taught me that uh things can be just perfectly fine as they are without having to change them.

Bob: Mm. Try these words just to see if they feel true to you, "Thank you for the gifts you've given me."

Chris: Thank you for the gi-gg-gifts you've given me.

Giving Voice to Stuttering

As Chris naturally finishes this heartfelt expression of gratitude for Stuttering's "gifts," he glances to Bob, as if for a cue as to where to go next. Bob therefore gestures toward the empty chair, touching it with his hand, and inviting Chris to occupy it.

Bob: Do you want to come over here now, just to take this chair and to kind of loan Stuttering your own voice, and just respond to Chris. [Chris: Okay.] Does that feel appropriate?

Chris: Yeah (nodding slightly).

Bob: You wanna try that? [Chris switches seats to embody his stuttering]. So, Stuttering, Chris has been speaking here, from the heart, and I guess in a different way than you're used to hearing him. What do you want to say to him about his awareness of your relationship now?

Stuttering: II-I want to say that __I'm glad to ___finally be having this conversation. ___I'm glad that _you finally gave me aaa-a voice. Um [Bob: hm], I've . . . I feel like I've always been treated as um . . . something eh-eh-*outside of _ww-who you are*. Every time you had any sort of an accomplishment due to your other charac-characteristics, you would *embrace* them, whether that was through your grades in school or through your aa-athletic aa-ach-chi-chi-chievments, every other part of you, you seemed to love and embrace and I was always *pushed to the outside* and um tried trrr-ried to bb-be *hidden* and anytime anybody tried to talk about me, whether it was your parents or anybody who wanted to, quote unquote, "help" you, you wouldn't even bring me up, you would, you would get angry and not want to talk about me. Um. . . .

Bob: Tell him how that made you *feel* to be so silenced and segregated.

Stuttering: It made me feel like . . . my whole being wasn't, www-whole being was negative. I-I felt like an *outcast*. I felt like a child whose parents didn't want him. Um, and . . . even when I would, ___I would show myself while you were trying to speak, your response ti-ti-ti-to me wasn't just to let me out, you would try to *suppress* me. And then both of us __would struggle because you would be *stuck*, _blocking on a sound so I wouldn't be getting out and you also wouldn't be sss-speaking. Um and that's not how it hhh-had to be. Um, I could have been right there with you the ennn-ennn-en-entire time and th-things didn't have to be the struggle that they were.

Bob: Tell him how you want to be with him.

Stuttering: I want to be with you just like any other part of you is with you. When you meet somebody aaa-at a bus stop you don't think about how tall you are or the ccc-color of your hair or th-the shshsh-shape of your shoulders or what your aptitude in any sort of ac-aca-acc-academics is. You just sort of speak to them; hhh-however, I'm always on your mind and I would like to be as ff-fully integrated into you as every other part of you is. Um, I don't want you worrying aaaa-about me any more than yy-you want to be worrying about me. I just want to kkkk-ka-*coexist peacefully* with you.

Bob: Mm. (long pause) Do you want to come back over here? [gesturing to the original chair as Chris makes the switch] Is there anything you would like to say, Chris, to Stuttering about this, this bid for a kind of peaceable coexistence and to be treated like any other characteristic?

Chris: Yeah, (looking at the Stuttering's chair) I want y-you to know that I hh-hear you and that _I've really been trying t-to make that change. Um, and I feel like over th-the years . . . that, aa-at the pp-present time it's the first time that, in the majority of our speaking situations, that hh-has been the case: where you are just another part of me and I don't think about you. I just talk and when I stutter, I-I-I-I stutter, and there's no tension, and, th___the words just come out even if they're ´d__disfluent. However, sometimes you catch me by surprise and I-I react in my old hhhhhh-habitual ways and um, I want yy-you to know that I'm not doing it on purpose. And that I'm really working on it. And it's, but it's gonna take time, because as we get further into this journey and the occurrences of that happening get lllll-less and less, we have __we have less time to practice it and as it catches us by surprise, um, those very ff-few instances are the only times we have ti-ti-to-ti-ti-t-ti-ti-to work on it. [Bob: mm] Um, and then by the time that we realize, "Oh, that was a time we should have been working on that," it's ti-ti-too late. Um, so I guess what I'm asking for is, is your patience, and hopefully we can get this done.

Bob: Mmm. Do you sense there's anything more that Stuttering wants to say about this, or does it feel like the conversation has reached a natural pausing place here?

Chris: (pauses in thought) I think that SSS-Stuttering understands that this is a process. [Looking almost fondly at Stuttering's chair, with a slight smile] He's been there the whole time too and he realizes that this is a journey. Um. . . .

Processing the Chair Work

Taking a cue from Chris's pause and disinclination to shift back to Stuttering's chair, having completed this meaningful round of dialogue, Bob then proceeds to "un-stage" the chair work and reflect with Chris on the insights articulated, as a way of consolidating them and considering their implications.

Bob: So, so perhaps we could just chat a little bit [Chris: mhm] about the conversation that you've just had. And I— you can maybe see some of the moisture in my eyes—I was very moved by the, uh the *humanity* and the *openness* on both sides of the conversation. Um, and I was also just curious about what caught your attention? What, if anything, in this, was an interesting observation for you, as you went back and forth between the two positions?

Chris: Honestly, when we first started, when you first sss-suggested this, I was expecting lot more, aa-a lot more *anger* [looks at Stuttering's chair as if to seek agreement] [Bob: ah] on both sides. [Bob: ah] Um, and I was surprised __by the *lack* of anger, the lack of raw emotion. It seemed much more [Bob: yeah], much more *civil* [smiling at Stuttering's chair] than I was expecting the conversation to be!

Bob: (Laughing) Huh!

Chris: Um, I think that's a testament to how far the journey__ has come. I think if this was a couple of yy-years ago there would have been a lot more [Bob: yes] aaa-a lot more anger.

Bob: Yeah, so this had almost a quality of affirmation of the journey that you guys have been on together [Chris: mmhmm] across this stretch of time. And now as you look towards a future, it is a future that has a very different, uh, aspect to it than the future your past might have had planned for you.

Chris: Yeah. There was a time in my past when the only fff-future I could possibly imagine ww-was one where I ___had [looks at Stuttering's chair with a mixture of shame over past feelings and hope for a growing friendship] gotten *rid* of him because otherwise it was too _p too painful to even think about. [Bob: yeah] Um, so every ch-chi-chi-transition point in my life, when I thought about that point, I didn't have a stutter anymore. [Bob: uh-huh] When I was in high school and I thought about going to college: when I was in college I didn't have a stutter. When I was in college and I thought about going to grad school: I didn't have a stutter. [Bob: Right] But each and every time I h-hit that point, he was still right there with me (still glancing in fondness and friendship at Stuttering's chair, smiling).

Bob: Ah . . . I had this uh, *slight smile*, that uh flickered across my face when he was over there, talking about how, um, the two of you would be in a conversation together and you would be "*stuck*," and I had the idea of, uh, you're *sticking with him* and he's *sticking with you* [Chris: mmhmm], and that had kind of a funny quality of affirming the relationship, the way two friends "stick together."

Chris: Yeah [still looking at stuttering and smiling]. And I think that's all he's really asking for, is __just to be treated as a friend. Um . . . and not give him this sort of negative ontology really [Bob: yeah], like his whole being is negative. [Bob: yeah] It was sort of an inherent aaa-assumption about hi-him [Bob: mm mhm] that, "Oh, this is bad I have to get rid of it." [Bob: mm] I don't know that that is entirely my fault. I think that's inherent in sss-society about disability [Bob: yeah], um, but nonetheless, uh, I don't know that that was really fair to him [looking over at Stuttering as if to apologize].

Bob: Yeah . . . I almost had the image as you guys were kind of looking back—he said something about feeling like a disabled child or something—and I had, I had that image of how a hundred years ago, uh, people might have hidden a disabled child in the house and hardly acknowledged its existence. [Chris: mmhmm] And um that that is a kind of, a social discourse around disability, that produces that kind of imprisonment, um, and I thought it was striking how you tended to invoke that same idea here. [Chris: mm] And it's really nice to see you (smiling) guys both emerging into the light of day together!

Chris: Yeah, it, I think it speaks to, um [catches himself again looking at Stuttering and smiles] . . . It's really funny how I keep on looking back over at him (points to stuttering's chair) as if he's still there!

Bob [laughing]: Well, he's probably listening pretty closely, with a lot of interest in the conversation!

Chris: Yeah! It's really funny, like, I'm almost looking, like, I'm aaaa-almost lll almost lll-looking like *fondly* [Bob laughing] over at Stuttering in the chair.

Bob: Nice of you to *include* him, right?

Chris: Um, but, it's in_interesting, it's uh, I think it, I think that's a gg-good sign that um, that future can be more positive.

Bob: Yeah, it's been a great pleasure to talk with you here today about this.

Chris: Yeah, y-you too Bob.

Concluding Thoughts

Not infrequently, clients relate to their communication problems with a certain degree of *confusion*, as implied by the Latin root of this term, which implies being *"fused with"* the problem. In externalization in general, and chair work in particular, clients are instead invited to "de-fuse" from the disorder, to gain the clarity and perspective that comes from not only recognizing, but indeed performing, their relationship to it. The results can be eye-opening and sometimes transformative, laying the groundwork for a series of *reflection*, *action*, and *protest iMoments*, and in dialogues like Chris's conversation with Stuttering, profound *reconceptualization* of the relationship between the client and his or her communication problem. Clients are often surprised, as was Chris, by the outcome of this dialogue. We have found that chair work, therefore, provides a flexible and effective tool in the repertoire of the creative clinician, and hope that you will find it similarly useful in your own adaptive counseling with a broad range of clients looking to realign their relationships with their disorders.

Frequently Asked Questions

Q: What if clients slip into a third-person way of talking during the chair work, for example by saying to the counselor, "I guess I just need to find a better way of dealing with my anxiety than running away"?

A: In that case you simply direct them to restate this directly to the problem. "Try saying this: 'I need to find a better way to deal with you. I'm tired of running away from you.'" In other words, just turn the statement back into dialogue to help the conversation continue. Keep it short, and don't give an elaborate psycho-educational lecture on speaking in the first person: Just do it!

Q: But doesn't the client sometimes feel strange about talking directly to the disorder? It seems to me that people would be uncomfortable with this sort of thing, and maybe even feel that doing so is kind of crazy.

A: Actually, most clients already feel strange talking *about* their communication disorder, a topic they usually avoid, so talking directly *to* it might not seem all that much crazier! Once they've grasped the idea of externalizing language, chair work is just an extension of the same idea. What is more relevant is that the clinician is usually the one who feels anxious about introducing the method (or any other novel way or working), but once she or he gets accustomed to it and the two develop a trusting working alliance, the client usually follows along and "gets into it" surprisingly quickly.

Q: Okay. But sometimes clients must just say something like, "Uh, I don't really want to do that. I just don't know what that will accomplish." What then?

A: That does happen, about 5% of the time. When it does, gently give it a try anyway, prompting the client, "Try saying that directly to the problem. 'I don't want to talk to you. I don't think it will accomplish anything.'" Surprisingly, that's usually enough to prime the pump and get the conversation going. If the client still balks, don't push it, but instead simply ask, "Okay, so something about talking directly with the problem doesn't feel right to you. Do you have an idea about what might work better for you at this point?" In other words, just invite the client's collaboration in finding a different way forward. After all, that's why this toolkit section is well stocked with alternative methods, and you might well find yourself inventing your own!

Q: Got it. But in this sort of dialogue, do the voices ever get confused, like if the client is in the problem chair, and then responds in a way that sounds like her own voice? What do you do then?

A: Good question. You simply direct her back over to her own chair, and ask her to repeat the remark, directly to the problem. She might also elaborate on it, perhaps with your prompting. Then just ask her to take the problem's chair once again and respond. Usually clients enjoy the exchange once they get the hang of it, even if it sometimes touches on significant emotions. Like other forms of role-play (see Chapter 21 on *Experimenting with Experience*), chair work is a playful way of tackling a serious issue—gaining more empowerment in relation to the problem—while wearing the protective mask of make-believe. Used well, it can go far toward addressing adaptive goals in the counseling, while also renewing motivation to engage in the technical interventions that are an integral part of the overall treatment package.

References

Greenberg, L. S. (2010). *Emotion-focused psychotherapy*. Washington, DC: American Psychological Association.

Hermans, H., & Gieser, T. (Eds.). (2012). *Handbook on the dialogical self*. Cambridge, UK: Cambridge University Press.

Rowan, J. (2010). *Personification*. London, UK: Routledge.

23

PLAY THERAPY

Clients for Whom the Tool Is Appropriate

Although everyone may benefit from play therapy, it is especially appropriate for children ages 3 through 12 years old (Carmichael, 2006; Gil, 1991; Landreth; 2002; Schaefer, 1993). Teenagers and adults have also benefited from play therapy, and, in recent years, play therapy interventions have also been used with infants and toddlers (Schaefer et. al., 2008).

This tool may be used to facilitate or extend the use of externalizing language related to the problem (see Chapters 8 and 11 for more details about externalizing), and, therefore, may be particularly helpful with clients who are struggling with a self-image that is dominated by the problem or, conversely, clients who have tried to ignore the problem's influence in their life. Additionally, all types of play may be useful for helping children to express difficult concepts or feelings and emotions that they are hesitant to verbalize.

Materials Needed

Materials need include Play-Dough®, Slime, clay, sand, beads, and other tactile materials, as well as puppets, toy animals, dolls, and other toys.

Description

Play is a fun, enjoyable activity that can brighten one's outlook, expand self-expression and self-knowledge, and deepen a sense of self-actualization and self-efficacy. In addition, play can relieve feelings of stress and boredom, stimulate creative thinking and exploration, regulate emotions, and boost ego strength (Landreth, 2002). Finally, play allows people to practice skills and roles that might be too difficult or risky to enact in the real world (Russ, 2004).

Speech-language pathologists routinely incorporate play into speech and language therapy with children, and audiologists often use play audiometry to test the hearing of young children. With play therapy, play is used to facilitate interaction that addresses affective processes that might be involved with the child's communication or swallowing disorder. Clinicians strategically use play therapy to help children express what is troubling them related to their speech, language, hearing, or swallowing problem, encouraging them, for example, to act out difficult situations with puppets or create monsters from clay that represent the problem. Similarly, if children do not have the verbal language to express their thoughts and feelings (Gil, 1991), play therapy might be helpful in facilitating the expression of those feelings. Furthermore, the positive relationship that develops between clinician and child during play therapy sessions can provide a foundation for building the client–clinician alliance that has been shown to be critical to successful therapy (Moustakas, 1997; Norcross, 2011; Wampold, 2001).

Play therapy builds on the natural way that children learn about themselves and their relationships in the world around them (Axline, 1947; Carmichael, 2006; Landreth, 2002). Through play therapy, children can learn to communicate with others, express feelings, modify behavior, develop problem-solving skills, and learn a variety of ways of relating to others. Play provides a safe psychological distance from their problems and allows expression of thoughts and feelings appropriate to their development. Play therapy allows children to change the way they think about, feel toward, and resolve their concerns (Kaugars & Russ, 2001).

A wide range of research supports the effectiveness of play therapy with children experiencing a variety of social, emotional, behavioral, and learning problems. For example, Ray and Bratton (2010) reviewed 13 experimental, 4 quasi-experimental, and 8 evidentiary studies of play therapy with children and concluded that, overall, there is strong evidence to support the use of play therapy with children. Furthermore, meta-analytic reviews of over 100 play therapy outcome studies (Bratton, Ray, & Rhine, 2005; Leblanc & Ritchie, 2001) found that the overall treatment effect of play therapy ranges from moderate to highly positive, and that it is equally effective across age, gender, and presenting problem.

Cattanach (1992, 1994) described two kinds of play that could be useful in expanding a child's experiences. The first is *embodiment play*, which involves the child exploring the world through the senses and utilizes such items as Play-Dough®, Slime, clay, and other tactile materials that can be manipulated. Particularly for young children, embodiment play might provide a safe, enjoyable environment in which further exploration of their emotional reactions to their communication disorder can occur. The second is *progressive play*, which involves children discovering and exploring the world outside of themselves through the use of toys, dolls and other objects. Progressive play might be used to help children better understand the concept of "externalization" and to explore alternative stories.

Case Example

Jimmy, a 7-year-old boy who stutters, was presenting with high levels of fear and anxiety related to speaking situations at school. His speech-language pathologist, working from a constructivist counseling perspective, decided to try some play therapy to help Jimmy directly confront his fears. At the start of a session, the clinician and Jimmy talked about the difficult speaking situations that he finds himself in and how he feels at those times. Jimmy told the clinician that when he gets into those situations he gets afraid that he will stutter and get embarrassed and so he just avoids speaking. They agreed to try to think of this fear as a "monster" that they'd call

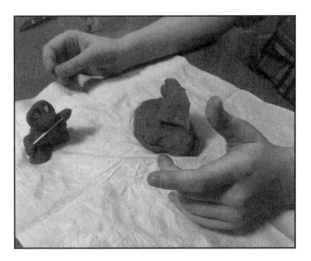

Figure 23–1. Creating Play-Dough® Models of Mr. Fear.

"Mr. Fear." The clinician then asked Jimmy some relative influence-type questions like, *"When you want to answer a question in class, what does Mr. Fear tell you that stops you from raising your hand?"* *"How does Mr. Fear get so powerful?"* And, *"What is Mr. Fear's kryptonite?"* Jimmy indicated that Mr. Fear gets power when he (Jimmy) stops talking and avoids difficult situations and, conversely, that Mr. Fear gets weaker when Jimmy stands up to him and doesn't back down. Jimmy and the clinician agreed that Mr. Fear is just a big bully and talked about ways that Jimmy could stand up to him.

Jimmy and the clinician came up with a few strategies that could help Jimmy stand up to Mr. Fear. They also created a set of Play-Dough® monsters that represented Mr. Fear—some big and powerful, others smaller (Figure 23–1). Each time Jimmy came to therapy, he would tell the clinician about a time that he used a strategy to stand up to Mr. Fear. If it was in a relatively easy situation, where Mr. Fear wasn't all that strong, Jimmy got to "smash" one of the small Play-Dough® monsters (Figure 23–2). If Jimmy stood up to Mr. Fear in a very difficult situation, where Mr. Fear was very powerful, he got to smash one of the big Play-Dough® monsters.

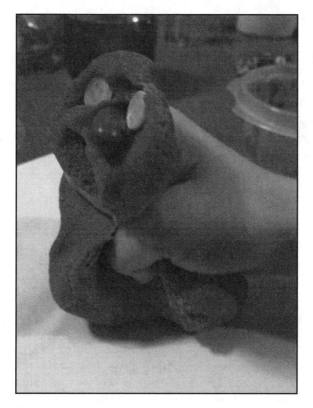

Figure 23–2. Crushing one of the Mr. Fear models.

Smashing the monsters was motivating for Jimmy, and he and the clinician had fun setting them up and deciding how they would get smashed! This action, however, also served to provide Jimmy with an increased sense of control and each time he smashed a monster served as a re-telling of an emerging story of Jimmy gaining the upper-hand over Mr. Fear.

Concluding Thoughts

In the hands of a creative clinician, play therapy can usefully extend children's expressive range for exploring the meaning of their communication disorders by providing any of a number of concrete media they can use to tell the story of their relationship to their difficulty, or to depict its influence on their social experience. But beyond storytelling, it also invites the *performance* of new narratives in which the child can cast him- or herself as a protagonist, either in the realistic context of the social world (e.g., depicting school or family scenes with dolls or figurines), or in the symbolic context of struggles against the externalized problem being treated. Such opportunities are inherently empowering, and as illustrated above can ally with technical treatment goals to reinforce therapeutic progress.

Frequently Asked Questions

Q: Speech-language pathologists almost always play with children as part of therapy, so how is this any different?

A: In many ways it is not any different at all. In fact, this is a great example of what we had talked about back in Chapter 1 where we indicated that counseling doesn't necessarily have to add onto what speech-language pathologists and audiologists already do; it is more about simply changing the way we think and the intended purpose of certain activities. In this case, the play that is already occurring in a speech therapy session can easily be adapted to incorporate some of the aspects of counseling that we discussed in the framework. For example, if a problem has been named, it is relatively easy to include externalizing language into a play activity in which some form of resistance to the problem is the focus, while still attending to speech or language targets that the child might be working on. Similarly, dolls or puppets might be used to act out scenarios in which the child must produce her or his speech or language goals but might also reflect a difficult communicative situation in which the child can experiment with different roles (e.g., assertive, passive, confident, etc.).

Q: Does the clinician play too, or just the child?

A: It might depend on the situation and the client, but, for the most part, clinicians want to take an active (rather than passive) role in therapy. Cattanach (1992) suggested that the role of the clinician in play therapy is to help the child use the play materials effectively, to play with the child, but at the child's direction, to be audience and empathic listener, and to record any stories or explanations about the play. These are important roles as the clinician is central in helping to give meaning to the play in the context of the problems that the child is facing.

References

Bratton, S., Ray, D., & Rhine, T. (2005). The efficacy of play therapy with children: A meta-analytic review of treatment outcomes. *Journal of Professional Psychology Research and Practice, 36*(4), 376-390.

Carmichael, K. D. (2006). *Play therapy: An introduction.* Glenview, IL: Prentice Hall.

Cattanach, A. (1992). *Play therapy with abused children.* London, UK: Jessica Kingsley.

Cattanach, A. (1994). *Where the sky meets the underworld.* London, UK: Jessica Kingsley.

Gil, E. (1991). *Healing power of play: Working with abused children.* New York, NY: The Guilford Press.

Kaugars, A., & Russ, S. (2001). Emotions in children's play and creative problem-solving. *Creativity Research Journal, 13*(2), 211-219.

Landreth, G. L. (2002). *Play therapy: The art of the relationship.* New York, NY: Brunner-Ruttledge.

LeBlanc, M., & Ritchie, M. (2001). A meta-analysis of play therapy outcomes. *Counseling Psychology Quarterly, 14,* 149-163.

Moustakas, C. (1997). *Relationship play therapy.* Northvale, NJ: Jason Aronson, Inc.

Norcross, J. C. (2011). *Psychotherapy relationships that work* (2nd ed.). New York, NY: Oxford University Press.

Ray, D. C., & Bratton, S. C. (2010). What the research shows about play therapy: Twenty-first century update. In J. N. Baggerly, D. C. Ray, & S. C. Bratton (Eds), *Child-centered play therapy research: The evidence base for effective practice* (pp. 3-36). Hoboken, NJ: John Wiley & Sons, Inc.

Russ, S. W. (2004). *In child development and psychotherapy.* Mahwah, NJ: Lawrence Erlbaum Associates, Publishers.

Schaefer, C. E. (1993). *The therapeutic power of play.* Northvale, NJ: Jason Aronson, Inc.

Schaefer, C.E., Kelly-Zion, S., McCormick, J., & Ohnogi, A. (2008). *Play therapy for very young children.* Lanham, MD: Jason Aronson.

Wampold, B. E. (2001). *The great psychotherapy debate: Models, methods, and findings.* Mahwah, NJ: Lawrence Erlbaum Associates.

24

THERAPEUTIC DOCUMENTS

Clients for Whom the Tool Is Appropriate

This tool is appropriate for children and adults of all ages (including clients and family members). It may be used to facilitate or extend the use of externalizing language related to the problem (see Chapters 8 and 11 for more details about externalizing), and, therefore, may be particularly helpful with clients who are struggling with a self-image that is dominated by the problem or, conversely, clients who have tried to ignore the problem's influence in their life. Additionally, this tool may be useful as one form of re-telling of the client's emerging preferred story. The tool is not recommended for children or adults who are seeking a brief consultation for a technical intervention, such as an audiological examination prior to fitting for a hearing aid.

Materials Needed

Therapeutic documents may take many forms. Consequently, the materials needed will depend on the form of the document produced. Basic writing and drawing implements may be used to hand-write documents or draw pictures that serve as documents.

In addition, computer software may be used to create letters, certificates, and posters that may also serve as therapeutic documents. Finally, if the document is in the form of an audio or video recording, some type of recording equipment (e.g., video camera, smart phone, digital recorder, etc.) will be needed, as well as a means for saving and delivering the recording (e.g., flash drive, recordable DVD, or email). Depending on the content and intended purpose of the document, it might also be posted to a social network such as Facebook or Instagram where it could be used to "sell" a clients' alternative story to people in her or his social network. Of course, the document should be shared with the client first and her or his permission obtained prior to sharing any document in such a way.

Description

The therapeutic document may be one of the simplest and yet most powerful tools at the disposal of clinicians. Fox (2003) reported on a number of informal client surveys that indicated that clients regard therapeutic documents as having as much impact as three to four face-to-face therapy sessions! The format and construction of these documents is exceptionally broad, with one primary consideration: they must be co-constructed (Payne, 2000). Fox suggested that one way of creating a co-constructed therapeutic document that reflects the happenings from a therapy sessions is to ask the client, "What was this conversation/session like for you?" Often, the client's response will indicate something like: "It was great, if only I would be able to remember it." This opens the door for the clinician to ask: "Well, what would you like to remember? Would it help if we wrote it down so that you can take it away with you?" From this point, the client and clinician can negotiate what form the document should take and what the content should be.

Therapeutic documents encapsulate new knowledge, perspectives, and preferred changes that have become part of the person's alternative but still emerging personal narrative. They may take many forms including letters, statements, certificates, creative writing, and audio and video recordings. Indeed, documentation can even take the form of clinician-written poetry that captures the key themes and images that percolate up from a counseling session (Neimeyer, 2012). Such documents may record specific happenings from a therapy session, but may also represent particular knowledge that the client needs to have available at times of crisis (e.g., difficult speaking or hearing environments/situations) or a way of spreading the news of preferred stories to others in the client's family or community.

Chen, Noosbond, and Bruce (1998) provide a detailed discussion about creating therapeutic documents and provide specific principles to "ensure that the document liberates rather than restricts, opens up rather than closes down, and constructs rather than subjugates clients' experiences of themselves" (p. 406). These principles closely follow the processes discussed in our constructivist counseling framework and include: (a) deconstructing the subjugated self, (b) searching for exceptions, (c) maintaining a "not-knowing" position, and (d) internalizing personal agency.

Deconstructing the Subjugated Self

The first principle uses language to deconstruct the negative self-concepts clients unknowingly have internalized. Many clients with communication and swallowing disorders can be profoundly affected by their problems and develop handicapped self-efficacy. When clients see problems as pathologies emerging from within themselves (i.e., a problem-person), they subjugate themselves and often feel blocked from acting on their resources. If clinicians are recruited into these subjugating views, they may not be able to help clients recognize their competency and use their resources to reconstruct a preferred identity. Therefore, it is crucial that clinicians write therapeutic documents in *de-pathologizing* language, reshaping the relationship that clients have with their problems.

To do this, clinicians should incorporate externalizing language into their documents. Therefore, clinicians should refer to the problem in terms of the name that they have agreed with the client to use when referring to the problem. For example, a client who has battled shame related to a profound acquired hearing loss might refer to the problem simply as "Shame" and, in the therapeutic document, the clinician might write about how the client *"outwitted Shame by being assertive and telling his Sunday School group that he had a hearing loss and needed to sit closer to the front of the class."* Similarly, a young client struggling with pragmatic language issues might name his problem "Outburst" and the clinician might write in a therapeutic document about how the client *"was able to resist Outburst on three occasions during class today"* and how he had *"developed strategies to make Outburst take his turn, just like everyone else."* In this way, clinicians can promote externalizing thinking that views problems as problems rather than people as problems and separates clients' identity from the problem, empowering them to take control over the it.

Searching for Exceptions

The second principle enlists clinicians to look for exceptions to clients' maladaptive patterns. In therapeutic documents, this may accomplished in two ways: (a) by identifying iMoments, and (b) by fostering the language of transition.

Identifying iMoments

As we have discussed in Chapters 8 and 10, iMoments reflect occasions when the client describes resisting the influence of the problem, dealing with the problem in some creative way, tapping into mostly forgotten personal resources, or even forgetting, for a brief moment, that the problem exists. Including iMoments that have been uncovered during the course of a session can provide powerful reinforcement for clients and help them begin to recognize previously unnoticed strengths and personal resources. Payne (2000), however, emphasized that therapeutic documents must be co-created and based on affirmed iMoments (what he refers to as "unique outcomes") rather than just "clues" to possible alternative storylines. What this means for the clinician is that the creation of therapeutic documents is either accomplished together with the client or the content of the document is based on an established (but, perhaps, still fragile) preferred story. For example, for a client who has been depressed about being on a pureed diet over Thanksgiving due to a swallowing disorder, the clinician might write, *"I was interested in your description of how you were able to enjoy Thanksgiving with your family despite your diet restrictions, describing how you even 'forgot' about your swallowing problem briefly during the day."*

Fostering the Language of Transition

In some circumstances, perhaps for clients who are making progress toward behaviorally changing a communication or swallowing problem, the clinician might include phrases that promote images of transition. Freeman and Lobovits (1993) advocated using phrases like, "dealing with an old friend you've grown out of" (p. 194), "growing out of a certain phase and moving into a new one," and "rising or climbing above" (p. 195) a problem. These phrases promote for the client an anticipation of movement that leaves the problem (or its influences) behind in a similar way to the "Dear John Letter" described in Chapter 18.

Maintaining a "Not-Knowing" Position

The third principle involves using language to maintain a *not-knowing position*. Recall that, as part of the constructivist counseling framework, we described how effective counseling takes place when the clinician gives up her or his "expert" status and defers to the expert knowledge of the client related to his or her problem and life (see Chapters 8 and 9). Similarly, in the construction of therapeutic documents, language that facilitates clients' self-knowledge usually stems from the clinicians' position of "not knowing" and is reflected in language that invites clients' reflexivities—"reflexivity" here refers to clients re-observing their own actions, perceptions, options, or meanings that shape their experiences—and honors their expertness in their own lives.

Consequently, in a therapeutic document, clinicians ask questions and make comments in ways that reflect their curiosity and sincere desire to learn. Rather than making assumptions about clients, clinicians ask wondering questions springing from a need to know more about what has been said or what is not known. This expression of curiosity about behaviors (particularly those behaviors that resist the influence of the problem) encourages clients to retrace the steps leading to positive results, thus increasing self-discovery. For example, referring back to the case of Mark, a young man who stutters but was beginning to gain some behavioral control (described in Chapters 2 and 9), a therapeutic document related to Mark's experience of being surprised by stuttering during a school meeting might include something like, *"I found it interesting that you were surprised by Stuttering's intrusion on your meeting the other day. I wonder what that says to you about how you are changing and who you are as a speaker?"*

Internalizing Personal Agency

Finally, the fourth principle is focused on ways to internalize clients' sense of personal agency. This might be accomplished by helping clients to view their actions as meaningful and effective in relation to the problem. For example, suppose a clinician is working with a client with moderate aphasia who is depressed because he feels ashamed that he hides from his problem by creatively avoiding situations in which he has to do much talking, always finding someone to talk for him or a good reason for not being the one to talk. This clinician might write something like, *"You seem to show a lot of creativity and resourcefulness in finding ways to cope with your communication difficulties."* Of course, the goal here is not necessarily to "buy into" the solutions that the client has been using but the *strengths* and *resources* that he or she has demonstrated that might become part of their alternative story and put to use in reconstructing a preferred identity.

Case Example

Charles and Anita brought their son, Josh, to get evaluated because they were concerned that he was not talking. Josh seemed to be

developing typically in all areas except speech, where he was lag-
ging behind. At 26 months, his vocabulary consisted of only two
words and he got most of his needs met by pointing and gesturing. Testing ruled out both a hearing loss and childhood apraxia of
speech, but Charles and Anita were very concerned that there was
something seriously wrong with Josh. This had been suggested by
Josh's grandmother (Charles' mother) who had been visiting recently and told Anita that Josh's communication was not normal
and could be a sign of autism, a growing problem for children born
to older parents. (Both Charles and Anita were in their late forties
when Josh was born.)

Initial observations of Charles and Anita interacting with Josh
provided a number of possible reasons for Josh's slow speech development that did not include more serious issues such as autism.
Primarily, Charles and Anita were very passive in their interactions
with Josh; neither parent played with Josh on the floor, preferring
instead to remain seated at the table in the therapy room. In addition, when talking with Josh, Charles and Anita both almost exclusively used questions, for example asking, "What is this, Josh?" and,
showing him a picture of a dog, "What does the dog say, Josh?"
When Josh wanted something, he pointed, sometimes making a
noise. Both Charles and Anita quickly responded to Josh's requests.

When we discussed these observations with Charles and
Anita, they acknowledged that this was their typical behavior at
home. They explained that they had always enjoyed their quiet life
together, often spending long periods of time reading or engaging
in artistic hobbies. When they decided to have a baby, they knew
that there would be less of the "quiet time" but they had agreed to
try to preserve as much of it as possible. They reported being quite
pleasantly surprised by how quiet Josh had been as a baby and how
he would play alone in his crib and seem quite happy. When we
suggested that Charles and Anita might want to start playing more
interactively with Josh, getting down on the floor and playing with
the toys with him, they were both very hesitant. "That's just not us.
I don't know if we can do that."

We asked Charles and Anita if they would be willing to try to
experiment with some different types of interactions with Josh. We
encouraged them to reduce the number of questions they asked

From: Anthony DiLollo
Sent: Saturday, November 05, 2011 2:35 PM
To: Conrad, Charles
Subject: Josh

Dear Mr. and Mrs. Conrad,

What fun we had in speech today! The two of you and Josh seem
to be having a lot of fun playing with the blocks. He really
loves it when you build a tall tower and then knock it down.
And when you, Mr. Conrad, tickled him with the soft bear – he
just kept coming back for more! You guys seem to "naturals"
at playing! I also really like the way you both were using
the description and parallel talk that we practiced, and how
you avoided asking a lot of questions, too. I think it is
really helping Josh to improve his communication.

I found your comments following the video clips of the
session very interesting. Did it really surprise you that you
could have this kind of fun with Josh? I wonder how it
changes the way you think about yourselves as parents,
knowing that you can do this and enjoy it?

I look forward to seeing you all next week and finding more
fun things to do with Josh!

Sincerely,
Anthony DiLollo

Figure 24–1. E-mail to Mr. and Mrs. Conrad that served as a therapeutic document.

Josh (unless they were essential ones like, "Are you wet?") and we taught them to use three techniques of indirect language stimulation: *description* (making a short sentence about objects that Josh had or saw); *parallel talk* (describing an action that Josh was doing); and *expansion* (repeat and expand on an utterance by Josh without asking a question). Initially, Charles and Anita were hesitant and unsure of what to do. After some modeling from the clinicians, they began to interact with Josh and attempted to use some of the language stimulation techniques they had been taught. By the end of the second session, we noted two examples of Charles and Anita playing with Josh and appearing to have fun, while using the language stimulation techniques. Before they went home, we used our recording of the session as a *therapeutic document* by showing them clips of the recorded session where they were having fun playing with Josh on the floor of the therapy room. We asked them to talk about the clips and how it felt playing with Josh. We then followed up with another therapeutic document: an e-mail that we sent to Charles and Anita, describing the *action iMoments* that occurred during the session (Figure 24-1).

As Charles and Anita became more comfortable with the types of interactions that Josh needed from them, we set up "homework" for them to use indirect language stimulation in daily activities (playtime, bath time, meals, dressing) and requested a total of at least 30 minutes of stimulation each day, gradually raising it to 45 minutes and then 1 hour. Three months after the first visit, at 29 months, Josh was re-evaluated and found to be using two- and three-word phrases, with an average utterance length of close to three words, which is within age appropriate limits. More significantly, Charles and Anita had a very different interaction style with Josh that included a lot more interactive play, with none of the hesitancy that characterized their earlier interactions. Before dismissing Josh from therapy, we presented Charles and Anita with another therapeutic document in the form of a certificate that emphasized their emerging story of being more interactive and having fun with Josh (Figure 24-2).

Concluding Thoughts

The use of therapeutic documents by audiologists and speech-language pathologists should be very natural, as we commonly correspond with clients in many ways and for many reasons. As with other aspects of counseling that we have discussed in this book, using therapeutic documents with clients is more of a change in focus and purpose rather than an additional aspect of our therapeutic interactions.

Certificate

This is to certify that

Charles and Anita Conrad

Have graduated from the
School of Having Fun

They accomplished this by:
Getting down on the floor and playing with Josh
Thinking about new ways to have fun with Josh
Knocking down tall towers
Getting friendly with Tickle Bear
Making silly noises
And
Laughing a whole lot!

This certificate gives them the right to have fun
whenever and wherever they want.

Signed: *Anthony DiLollo*
Principal
School of Having Fun

Figure 24–2. Certificate given to Mr. and Mrs. Conrad as a therapeutic document.

Therapeutic documents can be powerful tools and, as reported earlier, can have as much impact as three to four face-to-face therapy sessions, and can have an impact on the client long after therapy has been discontinued.

Frequently Asked Questions

Q: The idea of certificates and posters sounds great for kids, but do adult clients really want a "certificate"?

A: Actually, you might be surprised at how many adult clients respond to receiving a certificate. Typically, the certificate is meant as a fun way of retelling the emerging story and focusing on iMoments that are meaningful to the client. Many adult clients appreciate the lighter tone of a certificate as opposed to a more serious letter or email. Of course, you have to judge the needs and preferences of each client individually. As you get to know your client and understand the way he or she reacts, you should have a good feel for what type of therapeutic document he or she might prefer. Also, as in the case presented above, there may be opportunities to use multiple therapeutic documents that might be of different types (e.g., video, e-mail, certificate, handwritten letter, etc.).

References

Chen, M., Noosbond, J. P., & Bruce, M. A. (1998). Therapeutic document in group counseling: An active change agent. *Journal of Counseling & Development, 76,* 404–411.

Fox, H. (2003). Using therapeutic documents: A review. *International Journal of Narrative Therapy and Community Work, 4,* 25–35.

Freeman, J. C., & Lobovits, D. (1993). The turtle with wings. In S. Friedman (Ed.), *The new language of change* (pp. 188–225). New York, NY: Guilford.

Neimeyer, R. A. (2012). The poetics of practice: Becoming "well versed" in loss and grief. In M. F. Hoyt (Ed.), *Therapist stories of inspiration, passion, and renewal* (pp. 206–213). New York, NY: Routledge.

Payne, M. (2000). *Narrative therapy: An introduction for counsellors.* Thousand Oaks, CA: Sage.

25

MINDFULNESS

Chris Constantino, Robert A. Neimeyer, and Anthony DiLollo

You can observe a lot just by watching.
Yogi Berra

Clients for Whom the Tool Is Appropriate

Mindfulness is appropriate for a broad range of adult clients with communication disorders, and indeed is commonly welcomed by them precisely because it does not require communication, except perhaps with oneself. The practice of mindfulness may be a useful intervention in itself, as it has been demonstrated to relieve anxiety regarding social situations, but it can also contribute to the goals of many of the other methods addressed in this book, such as separating the self from the symptom or problem, enhancing externalization, or facilitating "experimenting with experience" with less emotional reactivity. Finally, brief intervals of shared mindfulness between clinician and client at the outset of a session can contribute clarity and openness to the session that follows once both members of the counseling dyad have mastered the basic skills of meditation. Sessions might then open with a simple establishment of mindfulness for a few minutes to "clear the space" for counseling, perhaps focusing on the question: *"What deserves attention today?"*

Materials Needed

Few specialized tools are needed for mindfulness practice beyond a cushion for sitting (or a comfortable chair), a quiet room, and perhaps a timer (especially for beginners).

Description

Therapy for people with communication disorders lends itself to multifaceted approaches. Our clients have physical impairments that restrict their ability to participate in the activities that give their lives meaning and purpose. Parallel to these difficulties are their struggles with meaning. Narrative constructivist psychology sees meaning-making as a result of our own personal construct systems, which are always already situated in historical, social, and cultural discourses. These discourses co-create these constructs with us and it is this broader socio-cultural context that gives meaning to our constructs. People with communication disorders are not only struggling with their physical impairments (e.g., hearing loss, dysarthria) but also with how they make meaning of these impairments and how their broader sociocultural context, of which they are a part, makes meaning of these impairments.

Our task, as clinicians, is to join with our clients in helping them co-create the life they would like to live. The journeys our clients are on are difficult, sometimes even overwhelming. They may not only be challenged to alter their physical behaviors by our technical interventions, but they may also be challenged to change their mental behaviors and their ways of making meaning by our adaptive counseling. In both cases, therapy can be quite the adventure!

We will be asking many of our clients with developmental disorders (e.g., developmental stuttering) to change behaviors and thought patterns that have become automatic and reflexive over their years with the disorder. These ways of being may be the only ones our clients have ever known; these ways of being have become so familiar that they have fused with the concept of self. Likewise, our clients with acquired disorders (e.g., dysarthria or aphasia) have had their ways of existing in the world dramatically, sometimes violently, changed. Their old automatic behaviors and thought patterns no longer serve them like they used to. Their concept of self has been damaged. They seek to develop new ways of being that will maximize their lived experience.

A concept called *mindfulness* can help our clients create the space they need to distance their concepts of self from their communication disorders. Mindfulness can be defined as "an enhanced attention to and awareness of current experience or present reality" (Brown & Ryan, 2003, p. 822). Mindfulness is not a technique as much as it is a quality of consciousness. Cultivation of mindfulness enhances attention and awareness of the present. To be mindful is to be able to recognize the reality of what is happening in the present moment with minimal conditioned reactions or judgments and with maximum vividness. Clients who cultivate mindfulness will be better able to detect and change reflexive thoughts, emotions, and sensations. Consequently, mindfulness can be thought of as a supplementary exercise that can be used to enhance more directed therapeutic work, and is especially congenial as an adjunct to the externalizing and reflective methods described elsewhere in this book.

More vivid awareness of the present moment can help individuals free themselves from reflexive thoughts, behaviors, and habits. Disengagement from automatic thoughts is useful in any chronic condition (e.g., hearing loss, aphasia, dysarthria, apraxia of speech, stuttering, cognitive communication disorders) in which feelings of inadequacy, embarrassment, shame, and stigma can be present. The individual can also be uncoupled from the reflexive avoidance that often accompanies these disorders (e.g., avoidance of speaking situations in aphasia or avoidance of moments of stuttering) through cultivation of mindfulness. The rich awareness that mindfulness brings to sensory feedback can facilitate more flexible responses and behaviors for individuals relearning sensorimotor patterns (e.g. dysarthria, stuttering, apraxia of speech).

Training in mindfulness allows individuals to remain in the present moment without habitually reacting to it, facilitating the development of nonjudgmental awareness of the present. It is an experiential rather than intellectual exercise. There is no objective, nothing for the practitioner to figure out. To be mindful is to be aware of the experience of the present, aware of the fact that the *only thing we can possibly be aware of is the present moment*, as "it is the only time any of us ever has" (Kabat-Zinn, 2009, p. 29). There can be no suffering in the past or in the future; we suffer because of how we reflect on the past and anticipate the future in the present. Mindfulness helps disengage us from such ways of thinking.

Mindfulness in Therapy

Before we address how mindfulness would look in therapy, it is important to note that it is just as important for the clinician to be mindful as it is for the client. We need to be mindful of what our clients are trying to say and truly hear them. This means that we are

Table 25–1. The Mindfulness Framework

1. You are not your thoughts, feelings, behaviors, or emotions.
2. Thoughts, feelings, behaviors, and emotions do not represent truth.
3. Your thoughts, feelings, behaviors, emotions are neither good nor bad; they just are.
4. Thoughts, feelings, behaviors, and emotions do not need to be controlled or corrected.
5. All thoughts, feelings, behaviors, and emotions are temporary; they will pass.
6. Observe thoughts, feelings, behaviors, and emotions with an intense, child-like curiosity.

aware of our conditioned reactions to what our clients say. This is especially important in therapy with people with communication disorders. Communication is what connects us to others, to our loved ones, and to the rest of the world. It is this connection to others that people with communication disorders struggle to achieve, so it is vitally important that the clinician working with them be as fully attentive and undistracted as possible in interacting with them. The framework listed in Table 25–1 can be used by both clinician and client to foster a child-like curiosity and interest in a world that can otherwise be cold and isolating.

Case Example

Instead of a single case example, we will explore each part of this mindfulness framework and give examples of how they may guide counseling interactions.

You Are Not Your Thoughts, Feelings, Behaviors, or Emotions

Mindfulness offers a novel view of behaviors, thoughts, feelings, and emotions. It teaches us that these do not make up who we are. We are not our thoughts. Our emotions are simply emotions, nothing more and nothing less. This first point in the framework may seem tautological but is necessary for creating space between our selves and our thoughts, feelings, emotions, and behaviors. In the case of our clients, it can create a space between themselves and their disorders. A man with a hearing loss may feel anxious about attending a cocktail party, stating, "I am anxious." A mindful approach to this feeling of anxiety would transform this statement to, "I have noticed that I am feeling anxious." The individual is not his anxiety but he is mindfully aware that his body is experiencing anxiety. Noticing these experiences as just thoughts does not make them go away nor does it take away their meaning. However, it does open up a space that separates us from our thoughts. Within this space we have enough room to observe our thoughts, feelings, emotions, and behaviors. This is important because, whether we like it or not, we are going to have these experiences anyway!

Thoughts, Feelings, Behaviors, and Emotions Do Not Represent Truth

These phenomena are simply the firing of neurons, the workings of our minds. There is no reason to give them the benefit of the doubt. A woman with aphasia may think that she will not be able to introduce herself and hold conversations at a social function. If she takes her thoughts to be truth she may think, "I know I will not be able to hold a conversation. It will be embarrassing." However, she does not actually know this is a fact; she simply had the thought that it will happen. Treating this thought mindfully changes it to, "I am aware that I just had the thought that I will not be able to introduce myself. I also had the thought that not being able to introduce myself is embarrassing." This critical approach to thoughts, emotions, feelings, and behaviors can open up dialogue between client and clinician about the meaning of these thoughts and what can be done about them.

Your Thoughts, Feelings, Behaviors, Emotions Are Neither Good Nor Bad, They Just Are

The above examples do not represent incorrect or wrong ways of thinking. The man with a hearing loss was not wrong for being anxious just as the woman with aphasia was not wrong for thinking she would not be able to hold a conversation. When relating to experiences mindfully we are prompted to abandon value judgments. We are asked to just observe our experiences as they are without labeling them as good or bad. There is no way they ought to be other than the way they are. By relating to thoughts, feelings, emotions, and behaviors in this way, clients can decrease their reactivity to experiences, especially to difficult ones. A woman with a cognitive communication disorder secondary to right hemisphere damage may often become frustrated and angry about her difficulties with pragmatics and her trouble reading social cues. When the clinician and client are able to talk about these difficulties as they are, without adding value judgments, they will be more able to create a space in which to make change. And in cultivating mindfulness, the woman with the cognitive communication disorder will be less reactive when in the actual social situation.

Thoughts, Feelings, Behaviors, and Emotions Do Not Need to Be Controlled or Corrected

We do not have direct control over our minds. We cannot will ourselves to have certain feelings or emotions or to think certain thoughts. Such efforts to exert control often only make matters worse because it puts the blame on our own shoulders when we do not have the thoughts, feelings, emotions, or behaviors that we think we ought to. These can lead us down a path to guilt and shame. Over time, many of our reactions become reflexive and automatic and are not readily amenable to conscious control. This is okay. When we are working within a framework of mindfulness, our reactions do not need to be changed, just observed. For example, a boy who stutters might reflexively tighten his larynx in reaction to a moment of stuttering. This behavior may be so over-learned that he has a difficult time not doing it. In fact, exerting too much effort to stop this behavior may increase his muscle tension and create a more intense and longer lasting block. A mindful approach would advocate entering the moment of stuttering as usual. The boy can be instructed to observe the automatic tightening of his vocal folds. Suggest that he not fight the tension, just notice it. Have him notice subtle details about the experience. Ask him where the tension is. What does it feel like? What happens when he tries to move on to the next syllable? What thoughts is he having while stuck in the block? Does any panic arise? Have him go toward this panic. Have him take "a good look around hell" (Santorelli, 1999, p. 88). What does he observe? These thoughts and the panic are neither good nor bad, they simply are. Have the boy contact these thoughts and feelings of panic, notice them, and then let them go. Letting go does not mean denying or suppressing. It simply means recognizing them without attaching to them, letting them float on by and change naturally into whatever comes next.

All Thoughts, Feelings, Behaviors, and Emotions Are Temporary; They Will Pass

The laryngeal block that the boy who stutters (from our example) is experiencing will not last forever, even though it may feel like it will. No behavior lasts forever. Neither do thoughts, feelings, or emotions. All of these are impermanent or temporary. The Sufi proverb, "This too shall pass," sums up this concept nicely. Have the boy place his awareness on the phenomenon of interest, in this case the laryngeal block. He will soon realize that the block he is struggling with is not static; it is constantly changing. Ask the client to observe the changes. How does the intensity of the tension fluctuate? Does it stay in one spot or move around? Where does it go?

Observe Thoughts, Feelings, Behaviors, and Emotions with an Intense, Child-Like Curiosity

Mindfulness gives people permission to explore their experiences with a newfound intensity and vividness. When viewing their experiences nonjudgmentally, from a distance, and without the need to control them, our clients can sit with them with a novel curiosity. It is this ability to sit with their suffering that opens up the space for real, long-lasting change. As our clients become more skilled observers of experience, they will begin to notice that no two behaviors, emotions, feelings, or thoughts are ever the same. Every present moment is unique and different from the moments of the past. Noticing this is, in fact, the genesis of *innovative moments* (iMoments), discussed previously in this book. Experimenting with experience, with a mindful eye for novelty, our clients can be cheered on to explore these differences with a child-like rigor. We can encourage them by asking how these experiences differ from those of the past. How are they similar? If Heraclitus were a clinician he might have said, "No person ever has the same experience twice."

Cultivating Mindfulness

There are several ways that mindfulness can be incorporated into therapy for communication disorders. As mentioned above, mindfulness is not a technique; it is a way of interacting with thoughts, feelings, behaviors, and emotions. It is most useful when the clinician and client are mutually mindful of the present moment and can create a space in which to observe these thoughts, feelings, behaviors, and emotions. Once a space is created, these thoughts and behaviors can be observed and engaged. Clients with newly acquired communication disorders will have a hard time engaging with their disabilities when their identities are wrapped up in the disorders (e.g., I am a stutterer; I am nearly deaf) and the resultant difficulties. By taking a step back, and untangling one's concept of self from the disorder (e.g., I am a person who on occasion stutters) the individual will be more comfortable making changes.

This distancing can be accomplished using the mindfulness framework described in Table 25-1. However it is not always easy to be mindful. Like any other skill, mindfulness requires practice. Mindfulness practice will not directly improve communication skills, but it will help to enhance other therapy techniques. For this reason, clients are encouraged to develop their own home practice. This allows time during therapy to focus on other activities. Many clients will find developing their own mindfulness practice to be challenging. Clinicians who have experience in developing their own practice will be better able to assist clients in developing theirs. You might also find it useful to photocopy the remainder of this chapter and share it with clients as a way of reinforcing your orientation to the method.

Just Sit

Mindfulness can be cultivated in a number of ways. One of the oldest and most widely used is through the use of sitting meditation. Sitting meditation involves taking time out of our day to simply sit and do nothing. During this time we have no goal, no objective. We are simply mindful of our thoughts. People often wonder how long and how frequently they should meditate. The obvious answer is to meditate for as long as you are comfortable; there is no need to overdo it. It is easiest to start with short sessions and as one gets more comfortable sitting, the time spent meditating can be increased. It would be reasonable to start meditating five minutes a day. Depending on time constraints this can be increased to 10 minutes, then 15, then 20. The length of time can keep increasing; it is not unusual for people to meditate for an hour. At the beginning, it will be best to pick a length of time and then set an alarm. As you become more experienced, you can just sit and stop whenever you like without the aid of the alarm. Typically people find it easiest to make time first thing in the morning or in the evening. However, evening practice can be hindered by drowsiness, so the morning is usually preferred. However, there is no "right time" to meditate; whenever is most convenient is best. This could even be five minutes in the office at lunch. Many recent publications talk about the benefits of mindfulness, but very few actually give instructions about how to go about cultivating it. Mindfulness is not a mystical or esoteric experience. All that is required is that you sit.

To start, find a quiet secluded spot where you are comfortable and will be left alone for the duration of the meditation. Sit down on a pillow or chair. If you are in a chair, sit with your feet firmly planted on the floor and your back straight. Sit towards the front edge of the chair so that your back is not supported by the chair's back. Cross your legs if you are sitting on a pillow. There are many ways to sit cross-legged, but the most stable is the most encouraged. The most stable position is to have your behind on the pillow and both your knees touching the floor. This can be achieved with the "Burmese" style of sitting (Figure 25–1) where contact with the floor is made from the knee to the ankle and one leg is parallel and anterior to the other. This position requires some flexibility but many people can achieve it with some practice. If you are ambitious (and flexible), the half and full lotus positions offer greater stability because your legs are "locked" in place and cannot move. However, these positions are difficult to achieve and are not necessary. Most people will do just fine with what Americans typically call "sitting Indian style". This is a cross- legged position where the ankle of one leg is underneath the knee of the other leg. Rest your hands in your lap or on your knees.

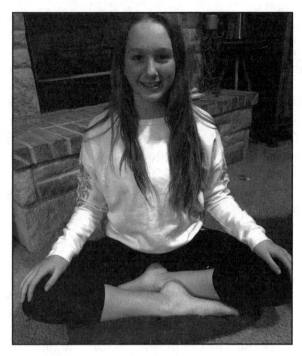

Figure 25–1. The "Burmese" style of sitting.

Focus on the Breath

Close your eyes. Now comes the hard part: focus your mind on your breath. Your breath, like everyone else's, occurs in cycles, inhalation—pause—exhalation—pause—inhalation—pause—exhalation and so on. Don't worry; this cycle will always be there, if you can't find it, then cultivating mindfulness is the least of your worries! Feel the breath flowing in and out of your body. It comes in through your nose, goes down your trachea into your lungs, filling your chest. Your chest then contracts and the breath travels back up your trachea and out through your nose. Find the spot on the most anterior aspect of your nose, right at the opening of your nostrils. This is what we will call your "home base." Try to feel the air passing by this point with each inhalation and each exhalation. You may not be able to physically feel the air here but you know it must pass this point. It can be helpful to visualize this abstractly. I like to think of a pair of saloon doors covering my nostrils that blow open and closed as the air rushes past. Others try to visualize the breath as a white mist flowing in and out of their home base. Regardless of how you decide to visualize your home base, focus your mind on it. Notice each inhalation. Notice each exhalation.

Some advice before we go further: Do not expect anything to happen. Treat the whole process as an experiment, an exploration into the present moment. Do not be anxious for results. Do not strain or strive for anything in particular. This is not about achieving a state of bliss or transcendence. The whole point is to watch what your mind does; to practice relating nonjudgmentally to the present moment. There is no hurry for anything to happen; take your time. Thoughts will come into your mind and thoughts will leave. Do not cling to or repress any of these thoughts. There is no need to attach to them or reject them. If a pleasant thought wanders into your consciousness, welcome it! If an unpleasant thought wanders into your conscious, welcome it! You are a host and your thoughts are guests. They have their own agenda; you cannot expect them to stay any longer or shorter than is in their nature. They each have their own personalities. Not all guests are pleasant and not all guests leave when we want. Of course we are not always able to remain indifferent to our guests; some may get on our nerves. They may aggravate us and even make us aggressive. No problem, this is just something new to be mindful of and observe. Notice what thought it was that upset you. Remember, there is no correct thought, no correct reaction. This is a practice of curiously and inquisitively investigating ourselves and our reactions.

Deal with Distractions

With this advice in mind, sit and focus on the breath. Your mind will wander. That is fine. Each time that you notice that your mind is no longer on the breath, gently, without judgment, return it to the breath. Remember, you did nothing wrong. The point is not to not have any thoughts. The point is to be mindful of the thoughts you are having. By noticing that your focus was no longer on your breath, you were mindful! Your mind will play all sorts of tricks.

It will wander about, distracting itself; this is sometimes called "monkey-mind". We do not judge our mind for its antics; it can't help it. These antics are neither good nor bad.

This process can be frustrating. Sometimes we just can't stop day-dreaming. Monkey-mind is acting up! The ideal solution is to try to be mindful of this restful energy and just observe it, but sometimes this is not enough. You may get so distracted that you feel like you are wasting your time. For those times counting your breathing works well to still the mind. They are plenty of ways to count. However regardless of the technique you choose, we recommend only counting as high as 10; remember we are supposed to be meditating, not counting. While breathing in count "one, one, one . . ." until the lungs are full, while breathing out count "two, two, two . . ." until the lungs are empty, and repeat. Another strategy is to try to count to ten rapidly on each inhalation and on each exhalation. You can also count each inhalation as one, followed by an exhalation as two or the combined inhalation and exhalation as one and then the next combined inhalation and exhalation as two. You can count any way you like. When your mind feels sufficiently calmed, stop counting and return to the breath.

Another obstacle to meditation is physical discomfort. Meditation should not be physically painful; however, at the start it could be uncomfortable. There will be an adjustment period during which you will get used to sitting. You might itch, your legs might fall asleep, and your back might hurt. Be mindful of your discomfort without judging it as good or bad. Notice it, be aware of it, but do not grasp it; simply let it pass. Remember, meditation "is an exercise in awareness, not in sadism" (Gunaratana, 1994, p. 62). Should pain persist then it is perfectly acceptable, even encouraged, to move until you are comfortable again. However, remain mindful of this movement. Move slowly and pay attention to what the pain does. Each new position you take will alter it; observe this change and watch as the pain subsides.

In addition to monkey mind and pain, you may also experience drowsiness. Meditation often produces a state of calm and relaxation. Most people live busy lives and only experience this sort of calm right before sleep. Unfortunately our bodies have been conditioned to associate the two. When you find this happening, observe what happens to your thought processes. Drowsiness has specific effects on your cognition; be mindful of these. This active, inquisitive response to drowsiness should negate it. If it does not, there may be a more physical cause of your drowsiness. Perhaps you just ate a big meal or did not sleep well the night before. Make a mental note of these things and try to meditate when you are most alert.

Concluding Thoughts

Mindfulness represents a way for clinicians and clients to relate to thoughts, behaviors, emotions, and feelings in a curious, nonjudgmental way. By focusing on mindfulness during counseling, clinicians can help clients distance themselves from their disorders and their conditioned, reflexive ways of being. This distance can give them the space they need to make the changes they desire. Mindfulness can be used simply as a way to relate to the world or it can be systematically practiced. Regardless of how it is used, it can be an insightful addition to other counseling techniques and behavioral approaches to change, and a valuable companion to the other reflective and active methods that comprise constructivist counseling for communication disorders.

Frequently Asked Questions

Q: Should we do sitting meditation during therapy sessions?
A: Brief intervals of shared or guided meditation during therapy can promote openness and facilitate communication during therapy sessions. It can be helpful to begin therapy in this way. However, these intervals should not make up the bulk of the session. Mindfulness is only a small part of the therapeutic process. Clients who would like more directed mindfulness training should be encouraged to develop their own home practice and to seek out mindfulness or meditation programs in their area. Clinicians also can offer separate sessions that are much more focused on mindfulness. For example, a group of interested clients could meet once a week with the clinician to meditate and practice mindfulness.

Mindfulness training lends itself to flexibility, and there are many options available.

Q: Is meditation awkward when it is first used?

A: It can be, as meditation is not something that most people are accustomed to. The idea of it is often accompanied by esoteric ideas of mysticism and transcendental experiences. This awkwardness is just something else to be mindful of! Both the clinician and client can pay attention to their initial feelings and reactions to meditating together. If clients are uncomfortable with mindfulness or meditation, it can be best to start out with very brief periods of meditation, as short as thirty seconds to a minute. Clients can be encouraged to try meditating at home first if they are uncomfortable with meditating in the therapy room. Remember, mindfulness is not for everybody, and our clients should not be expected to do anything they are uncomfortable with.

Q: Do I need to have my own home practice in order to use mindfulness in therapy?

A: No, the principles of mindfulness can be used even if clinicians do not have their own mindfulness practice. You do not need to meditate to use mindfulness in therapy. However, your own ability to be mindful will benefit from home practice. This does not mean you need to meditate every day, but some familiarity with the technique is helpful. Experience with mindfulness and meditation will also make you better able to assist your clients in their own home practices, should they run into trouble.

References

Brown, K. W., & Ryan, R. M. (2003). The benefits of being present: Mindfulness and its role in psychological well-being. *Journal of Personality and Social Psychology, 84*(4), 822.

Gunaratana, B. H. (1994). *Mindfulness in plain English*. Berkeley, CA: BodhiNet.

Kabat-Zinn, J. (2009). *Full catastrophe living: Using the wisdom of your body and mind to face stress, pain, and illness*. New York, NY: Delta.

Santorelli, S. (1999). *Heal thy self: Lessons on mindfulness in medicine*. New York, NY: Three Rivers Press.

Part V

PAYING IT FORWARD

The single chapter in Part V was designed with the college professor in mind and provides a rationale for teaching the constructivist counseling framework using a constructivist teaching philosophy and methods. A number of sample forms and activities to engage students in a constructive process of learning are included.

26

TEACHING THE CONSTRUCTIVIST COUNSELING FRAMEWORK TO STUDENTS IN SPEECH-LANGUAGE PATHOLOGY AND AUDIOLOGY

Tell me and I'll forget; show me and I may remember;
involve me and I'll understand.
Chinese Proverb

Teaching graduate students in speech-language pathology and audiology about counseling presents a number of unique challenges. First, most of the students in the class have little knowledge or experience with counseling. Second, many of the students (and, unfortunately, some of their supervisors) have "bought into" the myths about clinical practice that we discussed in Chapter 1, creating barriers to learning and implementing counseling in their practice. Third, we have found that most students fear "doing" counseling because of the abstract nature of the interaction and feel completely unprepared and overwhelmed. We hope the material in this book and the approach that material covers help to address these challenges. Finally, perhaps the primary challenge in teaching counseling is that the material itself—what needs to be taught—is not conducive to a lecture hall setting, meaning that a different approach to teaching is needed.

A Constructivist Approach to Teaching

Constructivism has roots in philosophy, psychology, sociology, and education and suggests that people construct their own understanding and knowledge of the world through experiences and reflecting on those experiences. As we learned in Chapter 5, George Kelly (1955/1991), in his *Theory of Personal Constructs*, suggested that people act as "scientists," continually using hypothesis testing to create meaning out of the stream of events they encounter. Thus, when we encounter an event, it is "tested" against our existing constructs (ideas/beliefs). If it fits, then the construct is "confirmed" and remains intact. If the experience is in contrast to the existing construct, the construct is questioned and may be discarded (usually only after repeated invalidation) or, alternatively, the event may dismissed as being irrelevant. This depiction of people suggests that we are *active creators* of our own knowledge.

Constructivist teaching, therefore, is based on the belief that learning occurs as students are actively involved in a process of meaning and knowledge construction as opposed to passively receiving information (Pelech & Pieper, 2010; Salmon, 2003). Learning always builds upon knowledge that a student already has (i.e., existing constructs), and students must be encouraged to use active techniques (e.g., experiments, real-world problem solving) to construct knowledge and reflect on, and talk about, what they are doing and how their understanding is changing. The role of the teacher, then, becomes one of understanding students' pre-existing constructs, guiding activities to address and then build on those constructs, and facilitating the students' reflection on the learning process. This contrasts sharply with the more traditional construction of teaching that casts the teacher as the "storehouse" and distributor of knowledge and the students as passive recipients of that knowledge.

Active Learning

So, what does this look like in a university classroom? Of course, there are potentially many different ways that someone might teach from this constructivist perspective, and we by no means presume to have *the* correct way; but, as of the writing of this book, we have, between us, six decades of experience teaching college students this approach. Typically, we make minimal use of teaching aids such as PowerPoint slides and course notes, but these are by no means taboo. Usually, however, we have found that such devices become distractions for students and encourage them to slip back into their "passive receptacle" mode. Of course, some students find this quite "distressing" and will complain that they are not being "given" enough information and, thus, are not being "taught" anything! Kelly (1958/2003) suggested that this is actually one of the primary roles of a university professor—to "teach our students how to replace certainty with uncertainty" (p. 296) and to teach them how to "live with uncertainty" (p. 297). Given the ambiguity of many of the problems clients will bring in for consultation, teaching students how to respond creatively and with confidence even in such circumstances seems to us to be a legitimate pedagogical goal.

Our classes usually follow a seminar type of format, with the professor introducing the topic and then turning the class over to the students to make comments and ask questions based on the readings that were assigned for that class. These discussions are facilitated by eliciting general reactions to the readings, presenting "what if" questions, pointing out confusing or perplexing aspects of the topic, and providing, and asking for, clinical and personal anecdotes and examples. This design fits with Kelly's (1958/2003) suggestions that university professors should be teaching students to ask questions rather than to give answers and to always be challenging them. We have found that this format encourages students to explore specific topics that are meaningful to their individual learning and that connect with their pre-existing knowledge and experiences, while also providing structure and guidance for students who are less familiar with such an active learning approach.

Understanding Student's Pre-existing Constructs

Getting students to share their thoughts about new topics is often challenging. In our classes, we use a couple of different techniques in an effort to elicit and understand students' pre-existing constructs related to class topics. One technique is to provide an open forum for students to ask questions, make observations, or tell stories that they feel might have some relationship to the class as a whole and the specific topic for that day. Students are encouraged to be creative and not to worry too much about getting us "off track." These times often evolve into lively discussions and frequently turn out to be reflective of students' pre-existing constructs.

Another technique that accesses students' pre-existing constructs, and forms one of the foundational aspects of the class, are the "reaction papers" that students write for each of the assigned readings in the course. Students are required to write a two-page reaction that reflects their personal response to the reading. In order to facilitate students' reflection, a format based on Kolb's experiential learning cycle (Kolb, 1984) is used. This format structures the reaction paper into three parts, *What? So what?* and *Now what?* (See Table 26–1 for instruction sheet.) The students are instructed that the "What?" section is to be simply a brief summary of the content of the reading and that this should be the *shortest* section of the paper. The "So What?" section is to reflect their thoughts, reactions, and questions related to the reading. This section is where most of the reflection and comparison to pre-existing constructs occurs. The "Now what?" section is to reflect how the student plans to

Table 26–1. Reaction Paper Format

What? So What? Now What? Format
This is a way to help you to get the most out of the reading you have done and purposefully reflect on how this information might improve your practice as a clinician.
What?
In this section, you will provide a brief summary of the main points of the reading (MAXIMUM of 2–3 paragraphs).
So What?
In this section, you discuss your PERSONAL reactions to the reading... connections to other knowledge or course material, changes in the way you think about the topic, connections to personal experiences, questions raised by the information, etc.
Now What?
In this section, you discuss the impact of this information on you (it can be personal or professional) . . . how it might change the things you do. This section might also include specific plans as to how you will incorporate this information into your personal and/or professional life.

implement what they have learned in both a clinical and personal context. (See Table 26-2 for a grading rubric for reaction papers.)

The students are informed that they should prepare their reaction papers prior to class and bring them to class as an aid to engaging in our discussion of the readings. These papers provide us with insight into each student's pre-existing constructs related to each topic that we cover and also help the students connect the new information with those pre-existing constructs as part of the learning process. Table 26-3 provides an example of a student's reaction paper, clearly written in the *What, So what, Now what* format, providing a brief summary of the topic, followed by a reflection on the topic with an attempt to create meaningful learning by applying it to an on-going clinical experience. She ends with further reflection on the topic and what it might mean to her as she moves forward in her clinical learning.

Table 26–2. Grading Rubric for Reaction Papers

	Grading Rubric for Reaction Papers (10 points)		
	2 Points/section	**1 Point/section**	**0 Points/section**
Format	Paper reflects the "What? So What? Now What?" format.	Some attempt to follow the "What? So What? Now What?" format.	No attempt to follow the "What? So What? Now What?" Format.
What?	Brief, accurate summary of the content of the reading (i.e., "What?" section should be the shortest section of the paper).	Accurate summary of the content of the reading but is too detailed (i.e., is the longest section of the paper).	Inadequate or inaccurate summary of the content of the reading.
So What?	Insightful reflection on the reading, including the student's thoughts, reactions, and questions related to prior understanding of and experiences with the topic (i.e., "So What?" section).	Basic comments on the reading that relate to student's reactions and questions but make no connection to prior understanding of and experiences with the topic.	No attempt to reflect on the reading or connect it with prior understanding of and experiences with the topic.
Now What?	Thoughtful indication of how the information from the reading might be applied now and/or in future practice (i.e., "Now What?" section).	Basic comment that the information from the reading will be useful/applied in future practice.	No attempt to connect the information from the reading to present or future practice.
Proof	Paper is printed and easily readable, with no spelling or major grammatical errors.	Paper is printed and easily readable, with a few minor spelling or grammatical errors.	Paper is handwritten or printing is not readable, or there are numerous spelling and/or grammatical errors.

Experimenting/Problem-Solving

For learning to be an active endeavor, students need to have the opportunity to experiment with different behaviors and to actively problem-solve in real-world situations. These types of activities help students connect with the material they are studying and process it as relevant to their goal of developing professional skills in speech-language pathology or audiology.

Role-playing counseling interactions in the classroom can provide opportunities for students to experiment with new behaviors. We use this technique to facilitate active learning and to allow students to "try out" techniques and interactions that we have discussed in class, without the pressure of dealing with real clients. These role playing activities are usually brief—10 minutes for each turn—and can take many different forms and have a variety of general and specific goals. Typically, after discussing a topic, students will then engage in a role-playing activity to experiment with the concepts and skills related to the topic. For example, a specific role-playing activity that follows a class discussion on externalizing would provide an opportunity for students to try out the tools of naming a problem and using externalizing language. Students can role play speech, language, and hearing scenarios (see the list at the end of the chapter for a wide variety of examples) or may use problems that they draw from their own personal and clinical experiences. Table 26–4 provides some additional examples of specific role-playing activities that might be useful when teaching a constructivist counseling class, which range from straightforward role plays of the kind discussed above to more complex enactments in the social world beyond the classroom. Instructors should ensure that at the end of each turn, students have the opportunity to talk about and reflect on their experiences, which usually takes the form of brief discussions within their pairs or groups, followed by a brief whole class discussion of what was learned by both the clinicians (i.e., what it was like to engage in the process) *and* the clients (i.e., what it was like to be on the "receiving end" of the process). Modeling the primacy we give to client narratives in counseling itself, we commonly invite "clients" to speak first about their experience, followed by observers (when present to the role-play), and

Table 26–3. Example Reaction Paper

Alexa

Reaction Paper #1

What?

This reading identifies the reality that a conceptual framework for counseling is essential for professionals to feel confident in their counseling abilities and that counseling is not just something to do with no context. Counseling is not a step-by-step procedure, but there are frameworks for helping professionals create a successful counseling experience. There are many approaches that can be used for counseling, but the one discussed in this paper was the constructivist theory. This theory takes from other theories like the personal construct theory and narrative therapy. Overall, the constructivist theory strives to put the focus on the person rather than the counselor. Letting the client be the expert, listening to personal narratives, using innovative moments, alternative ways on construing, and co-construction are five aspects of the constructivist theory that help one better understand the client and lead them to the solution.

So What?

One of the things that stood out to me was the "Clinician's Toolkit #2: Thin and Thick Descriptions." This section talks about how there is a tension between the "technical" intervention with the specific speech, language and hearing techniques versus knowing when one should incorporate a more person-centered counseling approach. There is also a difference in thick versus thin ways of looking at the problem. "Thin" questions look at the problem and are the general case history types of questions. "Thick" questions look more at the client's story and are better at looking at meaningful moments in the client's life. When I compare the thick versus the thin way of thinking and gathering information, I think of one of my clients who had a stroke. Because of the weakness on the right side of her body she does not like to write since it requires the use of her nondominant left hand. As an SLP, it might be easy for me to think, "writing is essential, you must be able to do it and that is why I am here to help you!" But after my first session, my client mentioned how much she hates to write and how difficult it is. When she writes, she is reminded of how much her life has changed since the stroke and that something as simple as writing is now a complex task. I am there to challenge and help her grow, but my perspective has changed slightly. Instead of going in with my technical attitude of fixing something or fixing a problem I see, I now try to understand why she doesn't like to write and how I can motivate her to do so. It's important to realize that only having a technical mindset will cause one to miss those emotions that may be affecting the client because of the problem. In addition, just asking the thin questions may miss the emotions behind the technical problem we see.

This doesn't mean I will never challenge her to try to write, but I can better motivate her now that I understand why this is difficult for her. If I hadn't explored deeper into why she doesn't like writing, I would have missed an important part of that clinician–client relationship. In some ways, the way I motivate her is like the "alternate ways of construing" aspect of the constructivist theory. When my client tells me she doesn't want to write, I usually say something like, "When you write you are working a whole new part of your brain you didn't work before and that's really beneficial!" I feel like this statement changes the way she thinks and suddenly puts her in control rather then letting the problem control her. I think that this example shows how as SLPs we will be using counseling and we will have to know how to deal with emotions that arise from the communication problems we are helping people with.

Now What?

I think it can be really easy to get wrapped up and almost be consumed by a fear of counseling. Not to say we shouldn't take the time to develop counseling skills and try to grow in that area, but I also feel like it is important not to be consumed by the fact that counseling is not a step-by-step process. I feel like one of the hardest things for me to grasp is that counseling is not a black and white area. There is not a series of steps that must be followed in order to reach a certain outcome. In addition, the reality is that everyone is different and that makes it impossible for there to be a step-by-step procedure for counseling.

Table 26–4. Role-Playing Activities

1. Don't ask: Find a partner and role-play a counseling session. Using a real problem usually works best. In this exercise, however, the counselor cannot ask any questions. (Hint: Focus on using minimal and direct encouragement, and paraphrasing. See Chapter 9.)

2. The Observer: Role-play a counseling session with a group of three, assigning one person to the counselor role, one to the client role, and one to an observer role. The observer notes questions to ask the counselor at the end of the session about why he or she asked something in a particular way or chose a particular type of question. This is intended to facilitate the counselor reflecting on his or her performance, but also benefits the other members of the group as the discussion of the session proceeds.

3. Experimenting with Experience: (See Chapter 21 for more detail on experimenting with experience.) Take on the role of a person with a communication disorder and play this role in public. Do this in a number of different settings and with different people. This can be done for most communication disorders. Practice in private (or classes) before going out in public is usually helpful, to attempt to be as authentic as possible.

Following these experiences, consider how it felt to be in this unfamiliar role. What fears and anxieties did this create? How might these experiences parallel those of clients: (a) who have the same disorder, and (b) who are trying to change their communication through therapy (i.e., also stepping into an unfamiliar role)?

finally "counselors," who can then reflect not only on their own experience, but also on what their partners in the role play have said.

Reflection on the Learning Process

Although active learning, experimenting, and problem-solving are integral parts of a constructivist approach to teaching, another important aspect is having the students reflect on and talk about what they are doing and how their understanding is changing. Class discussions and the previously described reaction papers can facilitate this aspect of constructivist learning.

One further activity that we have used to facilitate students' reflection on their learning involves students recording videos of role-played counseling sessions at the beginning and end of the semester. At the first class meeting, students are grouped into pairs or teams (depending on the size of the class) and instructed to create a 15 to 20-minute video of a role-played counseling session, with one student as the client and one as the counselor (and any others in support and technical roles). They are guided to try to use a real problem, but one that is suitable to be shared in front of the class. No instructions are given as to "how" to do the counseling, allowing students to display their initial knowledge/constructs about what counseling is.

At the end of the semester, students spend time reviewing their original video, with the goal of critiquing both structure and process and re-conceptualizing the client and the problem based on the constructivist-counseling framework. Groups then present their critique of the original session, using clips from the video and a reenactment of the session (a live role-play), demonstrating how the client and problem would be approached using the constructivist framework. The strength of this activity is that it encourages the students to reflect on what they have learned, forcing them to compare their previously held constructs about "counseling" (their initial video) to their newly emerging constructs centered on the constructivist framework.

Challenges to Enacting a Constructivist Approach to Teaching

Potentially the biggest challenge to enacting a constructivist approach to teaching is "letting go" of the control and the responsibility for students' learning—the equivalent of giving up the "expert" role as a clinician. From a constructivist perspective, students are the "experts" on their own learning and are the only ones capable of doing the learning. For many professors, used to the standard lecture-style classes, creating PowerPoint slides and course notes, and making sure that all of the information that the students need for their success is covered, the switch to a constructivist teaching style can cause anxiety, with concerns that something was left out or forgotten. Professors can also be challenged to give up the absolute predictability of the class environment that the "sage on the stage" role confers, instead becoming the "guide on the side," facilitating conversations more than dominating them. This means that the professors themselves have to become good listeners and conversation managers, in effect modeling the core relational skills that the aspiring clinicians in the classroom are striving to master.

Concluding Thoughts

As implied above, teaching counseling skills for working with communication disorders implies a rephrasing of the old dictum, "Those who can't do, teach." Viewed through a constructivist lens, "Those who can't do, *can't* teach," in the sense that experiential learning that closes the gap between theory and practice presupposes that the would-be instructor is equally comfortable with both domains. We hope that the present volume, grounded in narrative concepts, buttressed by a growing field of research, and replete with case-based presentations of usable skills and tools, supports your efforts to mentor and model adaptive counseling that supports personal change and reconstruction.

List of Speech-Language Pathology and Audiology Scenarios for Role Playing

1. You are a woman whose husband had a stroke. You are struggling to take on the role of "head of the house" and feel guilty when you make decisions without being able to consult with your husband (who has very limited communication).
2. You have a hyperfunctional voice disorder and require a change in the way you use your voice. You are a very outgoing person, who talks a lot and uses a louder than average voice. The voice you have been told to use is soft and breathy and it just doesn't feel right.
3. You have been diagnosed with laryngeal cancer and will shortly undergo a complete laryngectomy, which means

that you will no longer be able to produce any kind of voice.

4. You have recently undergone a complete laryngectomy and you are learning to use tracheoesophageal speech. Your spouse has reported that, despite being able to communicate effectively, you refuse to attend any social functions or do many of the things you used to do prior to the surgery.

5. You are a person who stutters and you have been in therapy for quite a while. The therapy has been successful in that you can effectively control your speech but it still requires great effort. You notice, however, that you feel very uncomfortable when using your speech controls when speaking to people who don't know that you stutter, kind of like you are deceiving them or tricking them into thinking you are a fluent speaker.

6. You had a stroke about a year ago and have been making good progress in speech therapy. Your speech and language are almost back to normal, but you still have some word finding difficulty at times. You also report that you avoid social situations because you are fearful that you will appear "stupid" when you have difficulty finding the right words to use in conversation.

7. You have come to see an audiologist because your spouse insisted that you need help with your hearing. You don't think you have any trouble; in fact, if people would just speak more clearly, you'd be fine. Of course, there have been times when you have noticed that you couldn't hear things very well, but you just put that down to noisy environments or just being a little tired . . . and the volume on the TV is clearly not working as well as it used to!

8. You have recently received a cochlear implant after spending most of your adult life with a profound hearing loss. The implant has been successful in that you can hear many sounds, including speech, and you can engage in "normal" vocalized conversations. You notice, however,

that you feel very uncomfortable when engaging in this type of interaction, kind of like you are deceiving people or tricking them into thinking you have "normal hearing."

9. You have been diagnosed with a moderate to severe hearing loss and have recently purchased hearing aids. The aids help with your hearing, fit well, and are comfortable. Despite this, you feel reluctant to wear them in public and they have remained in your drawer for the past two weeks.

10. You are the mother of a 4-year-old child who has had multiple medical problems from birth. The child displays no speech and has been referred by your pediatrician for a speech and language evaluation. Following the speech and language evaluation, the SLP reported that your child has almost age-appropriate receptive language and can produce some expressive language. You do not believe the report, as you know that you have to do everything for your child; you anticipate all his needs and wants and he rarely communicates with you beyond a few grunts and cries.

11. You are a college student who comes to speech therapy because you have difficulty pronouncing words correctly due to the effects of a speech problem you have had since early childhood. This has been a problem for you all your life and, now that you are in college, you find that you avoid social situations, asking or answering questions in class, and considering careers that would require you to speak to people. After the evaluation, the SLP tells you that you don't have any speech errors, but you find that very hard to believe.

12. You have a hearing loss and wear hearing aids. During an aural rehab program run by your audiologist, you discussed using strategies to improve your performance in difficult situations like restaurants and church, but you refuse to try them because you feel like you shouldn't have to ask others for help with your problem.

13. Your child has been diagnosed with a severe hearing loss but you don't believe it as she seems to react to noises sometimes and you think she is just a placid, quiet child.
14. You are an international student in the United States for college. You have a significant accent that many Americans find difficult to understand. You have been through some accent modification classes and have been trying to enact some of the changes that you've learned . . . but when you do this you feel awkward and afraid that you will be accused of "trying to sound like an American."
15. You have always had a problem with reading. Now, as an adult, you have become very good at avoiding situations in which your inability to read will be obvious. You have developed many strategies that enable you to accomplish your daily tasks without getting "found out." Doing this, however, makes you feel guilty, weak, and stupid—feeling that you can't tackle this problem but simply run away from it. Consequently, you don't believe that any therapy can help you.

References

Kelly, G. A. (1955/1991). *The psychology of personal constructs.* New York, NY: Routledge.

Kelly, G. A. (1958/2003). Teacher-student relations at university level. In F. Fransella (Ed.), *International handbook of personal construct psychology* (pp. 295–301). West Sussex, UK: John Wiley & Sons.

Kolb, D. A. (1984). *Experiential learning: Experience as a source of learning and development.* Upper Saddle River, NJ: Prentice Hall.

Pelech, J., & Pieper, G. (2010). *The comprehensive handbook of constructivist teaching: From theory to practice.* Charlotte, NC: IAP Information Age Publishing.

Salmon, P. (2003). A psychology for teachers. In F. Fransella (Ed.), *International handbook of personal construct psychology* (pp. 311–318). West Sussex, UK: John Wiley & Sons.

AUTHOR INDEX

SUBJECT INDEX

Note: Page numbers in **bold** reference non-text material.

thin and thick descriptions, 52,
96–99, 101–102, 109–125,
127, 129, 131, 172–173,
175, 184, **318**
Close-ended questions, 116
Clues, 99, 180, 284
Co-author, 78, 101–102. *See also*
Story: Re-visioning
Co-construction, 92, 101–102, 139,
184, 282–284
Cognitive anxiety scale, 73–74
Cognitive anxiety, 55, 73, 74, 76,
77, 97, 150
Cognitive behavioral therapy
(CBT), 241
Cognitive change, 25
Cognitive complexity, 74–76, 191
Cognitive errors, 54
Cognitive impairment, 227
Cognitive linguistic disorders, 255
Cognitive neuroscience, 48
Cognitive therapy, 54–55
Cognitive-communication disor-
ders, 239, 295
Combat veterans, 59, 62
Comfort zones, 37
Common factors model, 90
Community of concern, 68
Competencies, 34–42
diagnose the situation, 34–36,
39–40. *See also* Tempera-
ture: Challenges
intervene skillfully, 36–37,
40–41
energize others, 37, 41
manage self, 36, 40
Competing values, 40
Complex adaptive system, 32–33
Complexity science, 32
Compliance, 8
Conceptual framework, 92

Conceptual map of therapy, 103,
104, 159, **159**, 169, **169**,
179, **179**
Conditions of worth, 52
Conflict of interest, 26
Conflict, 49, 50
Congenital hearing loss, 239
Connectedness, 76
"Connoisseurs of experience," 59
Conscious deliberation, 48
Consciousness, 295
Construct systems, 63
Constructive alternativism, 60, 92,
97–99, 103, 240
Constructive revision, 58, 151
Constructivism, 28, 57–64, 69
Constructs, **59**, 61–64, 72, 136–
137, 312
and emotion, 63
as bipolar, 61
as reference axes, 62
core, 62, 136, 172–173, 180, 242
implied contrast, 62
peripheral, 62, 242
systems, 63, 72–76, 136, 240
Construing, 63, 73, 74
Content analysis, 73
Conversation, 17, 19, 20, 23, 27,
37, 41
Conversational effectiveness,
75–76
Core constructs, 62, 124, 136, 172,
179, 180, 242. *See also*
Constructs
Counseling,
counseling and psychotherapy,
18, 47
counseling as conversation, 16
counseling relationship, 9
definition, 17–18, 47
levels, 18

More Titles from Plural Publishing

Professional Writing in Speech-Language Pathology and Audiology, Second Edition
Robert Goldfarb, PhD, and Yula C. Serpanos, PhD

Telepractice in Speech-Language Pathology
K. Todd Houston, PhD, CCC-SLP, LSLS Cert. AVT

Professional Communication in Audiology
Virginia Ramachandran, AuD, PhD, and Brad A. Stach, PhD

Professional Communication in Speech-Language Pathology, Second Edition
A. Embry Burrus, MCD, CCC-SLP, and Laura B. Willis, MCD, CCC-SLP

Clinical Research Methods in Speech-Language Pathology and Audiology, Second Edition
David L. Irwin, PhD, CCC-SLP, Mary Pannbacker, PhD, CCC-SLP, and Norman J. Lass, PhD

Research in Communication Sciences and Disorders, Second Edition
Lauren K. Nelson, PhD

Workplace Skills and Professional Issues in Speech-Language Pathology
Betsy Partin Vinson, MMedSc, CCC-SLP

Narrative-Based Practice in Speech-Language Pathology
Jacqueline J. Hinckley, PhD

For more information, go to:
http://www.pluralpublishing.com